VEGETARIAN KETO DIET FOR BEGINNERS

A Detailed Cookbook with Delicious Recipes to Lose Weight Naturally with Tasty Seasonal Dishes and the Complete Guide to Always Stay Fit

RIHANNA SMITH

Vegetarian Keto Diet For Beginners

© Copyright 2020 by Rihanna Smith
All rights reserved.

This document is geared towards providing exact and reliable information with regards to the topic and issue covered. The publication is sold with the idea that the publisher is not required to render accounting, officially permitted, or otherwise, qualified services. If advice is necessary, legal or professional, a practiced individual in the profession should be ordered.

- From a Declaration of Principles which was accepted and approved equally by a Committee of the American Bar Association and a Committee of Publishers and Associations.

In no way is it legal to reproduce, duplicate, or transmit any part of this document in either electronic means or in printed format. Recording of this publication is strictly prohibited and any storage of this document is not allowed unless with written permission from the publisher. All rights reserved.

The information provided herein is stated to be truthful and consistent, in that any liability, in terms of inattention or otherwise, by any usage or abuse of any policies, processes, or directions contained within is the solitary and utter responsibility of the recipient reader. Under no circumstances will any legal responsibility or blame be held against the publisher for any reparation, damages, or monetary loss due to the information herein, either directly or indirectly.

Respective authors own all copyrights not held by the publisher.

The information herein is offered for informational purposes solely, and is universal as so. The presentation of the information is without contract or any type of guarantee assurance.
The trademarks that are used are without any consent, and the publication of the trademark is without permission or backing by the trademark owner. All trademarks and brands within this book are for clarifying purposes only and are the owned by the owners themselves, not affiliated with this document.

TABLE OF CONTENCT

INTRODUCTION **6**

CHAPTER 1. ...ADVANTAGE OF THE VEGETARIAN KETOGENIC DIET **13**

What Is A Vegetarian Ketogenic Diet? 13
The Advantages of the Vegetarian Keto Diet Over Other Diets 14
The Aspects of Vegetarian Ketogenic Diet 14
The Mistakes to Avoid 15
The Nutrients 16

CHAPTER 2. HOW TO GET STARTED **18**

Foods to Eat 19
Foods to Avoid 21

CHAPTER 3. A MEAL PLAN FOR YOUR FIRST MONTH **22**

CHAPTER 4. BREAKFAST RECIPES **25**

1. Coconut Porridge with Blackberries 25
2. Strawberry Chia Pudding 25
3. Raspberry Almond Smoothie 26
4. Vanilla Yogurt Pancakes 27
5. Broccoli Hash Browns 28
6. Sesame-Chia Bread 28
7. No-Bread Avocado Sandwich 29
8. Pear Oatmeal 30
9. Pumpkin Oatmeal 30
10. Veggie Burrito 31
11. Apple Steel Cut Oats 31
12. Tofu Casserole 32
13. Carrot Mix 33
14. Blueberries Oats 33
15. Apple and Pears Mix 34
16. Bell Pepper Oatmeal 34
17. Banana and Walnuts Oats 35
18. Simple Granola 35
19. Zucchini Oatmeal 36
20. Cranberry Coconut Quinoa 36
21. Gingerbread Porridge 37
22. Overnight Strawberry Cheesecake Porridge 37
23. Blueberry Quinoa Porridge 38
24. Blueberry Chia Pudding 39
25. Almond Flour Muffins 39

CHAPTER 5. LUNCH RECIPES **41**

26. Delish Carrots 41
27. Glazed Carrots 41
28. Sweet & Spicy Carrots 42
29. Bell Pepper Gumbo 43
30. Italian Bell Pepper Platter 43
31. Green Goddess Buddha Bowl 44
32. Cauliflower Rice and Mushroom Risotto . 45
33. Grilled Eggplant Roll-Ups 45
34. Eggplant Gratin with Feta Cheese 46
35. Tofu Pesto Zoodles 47

36. Cheesy Mushroom Pie 47
37. Meatless Florentine Pizza 49
38. Margherita Pizza with Cauliflower Crust 49
39. Almond Tofu Loaf 50
40. Kale and Mushroom Biryani 51
41. Mushroom Pizza Bowls with Avocado & Cilantro 52
42. Pistachios and Cheese Stuffed Zucchinis... 53
43. Soy Chorizo-Asparagus Bowl................... 54
44. Creamy Brussels Sprouts Bowls............... 54
45. Green Beans and Radishes Bake 55
46. Avocado and Radish Bowls...................... 55
47. Celery and Radish Soup 56
48. Lime Avocado and Cucumber Soup 56
49. Avocado and Kale Soup............................ 57
50. Spinach and Cucumber Salad 57

CHAPTER 6. SNACK RECIPES 58

51. Nori Snack Rolls....................................... 58
52. Risotto Bites.. 58
53. Jicama and Guacamole.............................. 59
54. Curried Tofu "Egg Salad" Pitas................ 60
55. Garden Patch Sandwiches on Multigrain Bread 60
56. Garden Salad Wraps.................................. 61
57. Black Sesame Wonton Chips.................... 62
58. Marinated Mushroom Wraps.................... 62
59. Tamari Toasted Almonds 63
60. Avocado and Tempeh Bacon Wraps......... 64
61. Kale Chips 64
62. Tempeh-Pimiento Cheese Ball 65
63. Seaweed Crackers 65

64. Sesame Tamari Almonds 66
65. Edamame Avocado Hummus 66
66. Pizza Cheese Ball 67
67. Tahini Keto Bagels.................................... 67
68. Zucchini Nests 68
.... 68
69. Low Carb Bibimbap 68
70. Walnut Carrot Bombs 69
71. Nutty Zucchini Salad................................. 70
72. Kale Pate Spread 70
73. Smoked Almonds....................................... 71
74. Roasted Garlic Mushrooms 71
75. Mediterranean Cucumber Bites 72

CHAPTER 7. DINNER RECIPES........................73

76. Seitan Tex-Mex Casserole 73
77. Avocado Coconut Pie................................ 74
.... 74
78. Baked Mushrooms with Creamy Brussels Sprouts 75
79. Pimiento Tofu balls................................... 76
80. Tempeh with Garlic Asparagus 76
81. Mushroom Curry Pie................................. 77
82. Spicy Cheese with Tofu Balls................... 78
83. Tempeh Coconut Curry Bake.................... 79
84. Kale and Mushroom Pierogis 80
85. Mushroom Lettuce Wraps 81
86. Tofu and Spinach Lasagna with Red Sauce 81
87. Green Avocado Carbonara........................ 83
88. Cashew Buttered Quesadillas with Leafy Greens 84

89.	Zucchini Boats with Vegan Cheese	85
90.	Tempeh Garam Masala Bake	85
91.	Caprese Casserole	86
92.	Lemon Garlic Mushrooms	87
93.	Almond Green Beans	87
94.	Fried Okra	88
95.	Super Healthy Beet Greens Salad	88
96.	Coconut Yogurt with Chia Seeds and Almonds	89
97.	Super Delicious Cucumber Salad	89
98.	Pudding Delight with Banana & Coconut	90
99.	Extra Easy Cheese Sandwich	90
100.	India Super Easy Summer Cooler	91

CHAPTER 8. DESSERT RECIPES 92

101.	Strawberry Coconut Parfait	92
102.	Lemon-Chocolate Truffles	92
103.	Blackberry and Red Wine Crumble	93
104.	Cinnamon-Chocolate Cake	94
105.	Himalayan Raspberry Fat Bombs	94
106.	Cashew-Chocolate Cheesecake	95
107.	Creamy Avocado Drink	96
108.	Raspberry Cookies	96
109.	Lenny & Larry's Cookies	97
110.	Zucchini Chocolate Brownies	97
111.	Fudgy Pumpkin Brownies	98
112.	Cinnamon Roll Bars	98
113.	Snickers Bars	99
114.	Lemon Coconut Crack Bars	99
115.	Gingerbread Cookie Bars	100
116.	Cocoa Berries Mousse	100
117.	Nutmeg Pudding	101
118.	Lime Cherries and Rice Pudding	101
119.	Chocolate Pudding	102
120.	Coffee and Rhubarb Cream	102
121.	Chocolate Sea Salt Almonds	103
122.	Salted Caramel Cashew Brittle	103
123.	Cookies and Cream Parfait	104
124.	Pecan Pie Pudding	104
125.	Chocolate Avocado Pudding	105

CONCLUSION 106

Introduction

In one form or another ketogenic, or keto, the diet has been in use for centuries. In ancient Greece, physicians treated various diseases, especially the disease of epilepsy, by making changes in their patient's diets. Many Greek physicians believed that there was a physical and rational basis to use dietary therapy to cure illnesses and conditions.

The first study of a modern type was not conducted until the twentieth century. A group of patients with epilepsy was treated with a vegetarian diet that was low in calories. Those who maintained strict adherence to the diet were able to greatly decrease or end their seizures. Scientists who studied the results of this experiment found that there were three compounds that are water soluble and are located in the liver of healthy people who were adhering to a very low calorie or a starvation diet. They coined the term 'ketone bodies' as a name to call these compounds. Other doctors built on this research and discovered that the body could be made to produce ketone bodies when it was fed a high fat low carbohydrate diet. Because of the ketone bodies, the term 'ketogenic' was first used.

The first keto diets varied widely in the ratio of fats to proteins consumed until a pediatrician tried using the diet on his patients to see if it could reduce or eliminate their symptoms of epilepsy. His formula was for the patient to consume only one gram of protein for every pound of body weight, fifteen to twenty grams of carbs per day, and the rest of the caloric intake would be made up of fat. Besides reducing the seizures of epilepsy doctors noted that their patients slept longer and more soundly, had an improved level of alertness, and experienced better overall behavior with very few or no side effects.

The keto diet was widely used as a treatment for epilepsy until the middle to the latter part of the twentieth century when anti-convulsing drugs became more readily available and highly popular. Taking a pill is much easier than sticking to a rigid diet. So, the keto diet fell out of favor until the 1990s, when a television producer and his wife were searching for a treatment for their young son, who suffered from debilitating seizures that even high doses of medicine did not stop. Their child did so well on the keto diet that they promoted it to everyone who would listen, and the diet was once again popular.

In normal physical processes, the human body will burn carbs for energy. The body turns carbs into sugar, or glucose, during the process of digestion.

When people eat the pancreas gets a signal from the brain to produce insulin to help take the sugar produced by digestion through the bloodstream and into the cells. The insulin is actually the key that gets the blood sugar into the cells. The pancreas will produce as much insulin as the body needs to transport and disperse the amount of blood sugar the body has to get rid of. The body will also store a precise amount of blood sugar in the liver in the form of glycogen. This is a type of emergency store in case the body faces starvation before the next meal appears.

The problem begins when there is too much blood sugar, as usually happens when people eat a high sugar high carb diet. Eventually, the cells will have all of the glucose that they need and they will begin to ignore the insulin when it comes knocking on the cell door. This is known as insulin resistance. The body then needs to find a place to put all of this excess glucose so it stores it as fat beginning around the organs of the abdomen and then spreading out to other areas of the body.

The predominant goal when following the keto diet is to lower the consumption of carbs enough to burn body fat enough to cause massive weight loss. The other part of that goal is to feel fewer food cravings, especially for sugary foods, while making the body feel full with less food consumed.

When the consumption of carbs is restricted to a low level the body needs to find a new source of energy for the cells to be able to function. The body will first begin to burn the glycogen that is stored in the liver when the supply of blood sugar in the bloodstream decreases. The liver can store enough glycogen to fuel the body for about forty-eight hours. After that time the body will search for other ways to obtain fuel for the body to use. The liver will use the stored fat in the body to break it down to make fuel.

Your body goes through a perfectly normal metabolic process called ketosis when it begins to burn stored fat for fuel. This is a perfectly normal process the body goes through when access to carbs is limited or eliminated. The body produces ketones when it goes into ketosis and this is what the body uses for fuel instead of carbs. This is a feature that was built into the body ages ago to keep early man from starving to death during times when food was not readily available.

Ketosis is the name given to the body's function of making ketones from stored fat for fuel for the body. The body will usually enter ketosis after about three or four days of eating a low carb diet. The main purpose of following the keto diet is to get the body to enter ketosis because this means the body has begun burning stored fat. Most people enter ketosis with few to no symptoms, and some people experience what is called the 'keto flu' because the symptoms feel much like having the flu.

During the beginning of ketosis, the person may experience very bad breath. This happens because the body is breaking down toxins with the breakdown of stored fat, and toxins are removed from the body in three ways—through urination, through sweating, and through the respiratory system.

So your body is sending out toxins with every exhale. This symptom will only last a few days, and more tooth brushing or use of mouthwash will help lessen the symptoms.

Also when going into ketosis you will probably feel less hungry. This is because the body is learning to use food more efficiently. This is also because carbs are digested quickly and leave you feeling hungry soon after eating them. And protein and fat take longer to digest, so you will feel less hungry than before.

The keto flu, like the flu that is brought on by a virus, can leave you feeling exhausted. Part of this is due to the decreased intake of carbs that give instant energy to the body. Part of this may be caused by slight dehydration.

Excess fat stored in the body holds water, which is why the first few pounds lost on any diet are water weight. You can combat this fatigue by drinking more water and by drinking sugar-free sports drinks with electrolytes.

And during the first few days of ketosis, you will likely see a decrease in your performance while exercising. While exercise is important to weight loss it might be necessary during this time to lessen the intensity of your workouts. Also, your muscles need time to become adjusted to the difference in the source of the fuel they are receiving.

Some people experience issues with the digestive system like diarrhea or constipation. Constipation is usually more of an issue that diarrhea is. Diarrhea comes from an increased intake of fat in the diet and your body will become used to the increase of fat in your diet. Constipation comes from not drinking enough water and from not eating enough vegetables. There are certain low carb veggies that are allowed on the keto diet and these should be eaten daily to keep your system regular.

Following a ketogenic plan should not be thought of as a diet plan but it should be viewed as a lifestyle change. This is a way of eating that can be done for many years. As long as you follow the keto diet you will continue to enjoy the benefits of the keto diet.

What is Ketogenic Diet?

Many people will shorten the ketogenic diet down and just call it a keto diet. This word was created because when you do this diet, your body will create small fuel molecules that are called ketones. These get used as an alternate source of fuel for our bodies. These get used when the body's glucose supplies get low.

When you don't eat a whole lot of carbs, these ketones are produced. This holds true when protein intake is kept at a moderate level. Eating too much protein can cause the body to turn it into sugar.

Your liver is able to create ketones from the fat your body has stored. The body then uses these ketones as fuel for many different parts of the body including the brain. Amazingly, the brain uses a lot of energy in just one day.

Low Carb

A keto diet is a very strict low carb diet. You are going to eat only 20 grams or less of net carbs each day.

When you have achieved your weight loss goals, you can begin to increase your carb intake. This needs to be done slowly so you don't gain the weight back.

Basics

This is a great diet, but there is a right and wrong way to do it. You have to begin this diet the right way so you will get faster and better results.

In theory, a keto diet is simple; low carbs, high fat. This isn't telling you what you can and can't eat. There is a list of complete foods you are allowed to eat, which we will discuss later. For now, here is a list of what you can eat:

- Heavy fats like tallow, olive oil, bacon fat, butter, lard, ghee, and coconut oil.
- Meats including organ meat.
- Eggs
- Fish and seafood
- Nonstarchy vegetables. All the leafy greens you want.
- Berries such as strawberries, blueberries, and raspberries.

Your typical day might look something like:

- Breakfast might include eggs and bacon.
- Lunch might be a chicken salad with a cup of bone broth.
- Dinner might be a steak with a side of veggies and a keto friendly dessert.

Some people like to snack between meals. If you are one of these people, some good choices are broth, cheese sticks, nuts, meat sticks, and celery sticks. You need to watch the number of snacks as these can make your total calorie count go up.

The keto diet is easy to personalize. You can experiment and find out what works best for you. Some people might realize they need more fat in their diet and others can eat fewer carbs. Some people even try intermittent fasting.

Many people who intermittent fast skip breakfast and will eat their first meat about one in the afternoon. This will up your ketosis power.

Macros

Macros have already been mentioned a few times. You are probably wondering by now what they are. Macros are short for macronutrients when used in the context of the keto diet.

Carbs are the only macro that you don't have to consume to stay alive. There are essential fatty and amino acids that are the building blocks of fats and proteins, but there aren't any essential carbs.

Carbs are made of two things: starch and sugar. Fiber is looked at as a carb, but with a keto diet, it isn't counted toward your total carb intake. Fiber isn't counted since the body doesn't digest fiber, so it doesn't have any effect on blood sugar.

When you look at a nutrition label, you need to first find the number of total carbs and then look for fiber. You are going to subtract the amount of fiber from the total number of carbs; this gives you the net carbs.

Total carbs – fiber = net carbs.

This just means that net carbohydrates only count the sugars and starches in the carbohydrates you eat.

In order for you to succeed, you need to find food that is naturally low in carbs and the ones that aren't. Not all foods are obvious. It is obvious that potatoes are high in carbs, but do you realize that bananas are also very high in carbs, too?

For anyone who is just beginning a keto diet, you need to try to consume about 20 grams of net carbs every day.

Protein is important for our bodies since it helps preserve lean muscle mass, the energy source in the absence of carbs makes hormones and enzymes, immune function, tissue repair, and growth. Protein plays an important role in biological processes. Proteins are the building blocks for healthy bodies.

When eaten, proteins are broken down into amino acids. Nine of these can't be produced by our bodies. This is why these essential amino acids need to come from foods. These nine include lysine, valine, threonine, histidine, isoleucine, tryptophan, leucine, phenylalanine, and methionine. If there is a deficiency in protein or any of these amino acids, it could cause malnutrition, kwashiorkor, or many other health problems.

When you are doing a keto diet, you have to be sure you are eating enough protein to preserve your lean body mass. The amount you consume, all depends on how much lean body mass you have now. Here is a guideline:

- .7 to .8 grams of protein per pound of muscle to help preserve your muscle mass.

- .8 to 1.2 grams of protein per pound of muscle to help you increase your muscle mass.

You don't want to lose any body mass, only gain or preserve it. Many people just focus on losing weight, but many times when people lose weight, they also lose muscle along with fat. Your goal needs to be losing weight while saving your muscle. This is important to keep up your metabolism.

The main thing is to make sure you don't get crazy when consuming protein when doing a keto diet. Too much might put too much stress on the kidneys and can affect ketosis. Try keeping your macros in the above ranges.

Here's an example:

Let's say you weigh 160 pounds and you have 30 percent body fat. This means you have about 48 pounds of body fat. Now you are going to subtract your body fat from your total weight and this gives you your lean body mass. For this, it would be 112 pounds.

In order to find the amount of protein you need to consume, you take the lean body mass number and multiply it by the ratio from earlier. In this example, you need to consume 89.6 grams of protein every day to preserve your muscle mass. It will look like this:

112 pounds muscle x .8 grams protein = 89.6 grams.

The last macro is fat. You need to consume the right amount of fat to maintain cell membranes, provide protective cushioning for organs, absorb certain vitamins, development, energy, and growth. These fats also help you feel fuller longer.

Dietary fat gets broken down into fatty acids and glycerol. The body can't synthesize two types of fatty acids, so it is important that you incorporate them into your diet. These fatty acids are linolenic acid and linoleic acid.

These facts are satiating, so it is perfect for people who want to fight off hunger pangs. You need to figure out how much fat you should eat. If your carbs are at a minimum, you have figured out how much protein you should eat, and then the rest of your dietary needs must be met with fat.

In order to maintain your weight, you are going to eat enough calories from fat in order to support your normal daily activities. If you want to burn fat, you need to eat in a deficit.

You have been given a lot of information to help you figure out your macros, but there are easier ways to figure this out. There are many online calculators that will figure these numbers without you getting a headache. If you would like to use an online calculator, check out this website: Ketogains. it works great.

If you would like to figure it out on your own, let's continue with the 160-pound example from above. Let's say this person is a female, stands 5'4", in her late 20s, and sits behind a desk all day. She is mainly sedentary.

Let's plug her into a calculator:

The base metabolic rate would be 1467 kcal.

Daily energy expenditure would be 1614 kcal.

She is going to need to consume about 90 grams of protein, 20 grams of net carbs, and 86 grams of fat. Her intake is 72 percent fat, 23 percent protein, and 5 percent carbs.

Now you know what macros are and how to find your numbers. You are on your way to beginning a ketogenic diet.

Advantage of the Vegetarian Ketogenic Diet

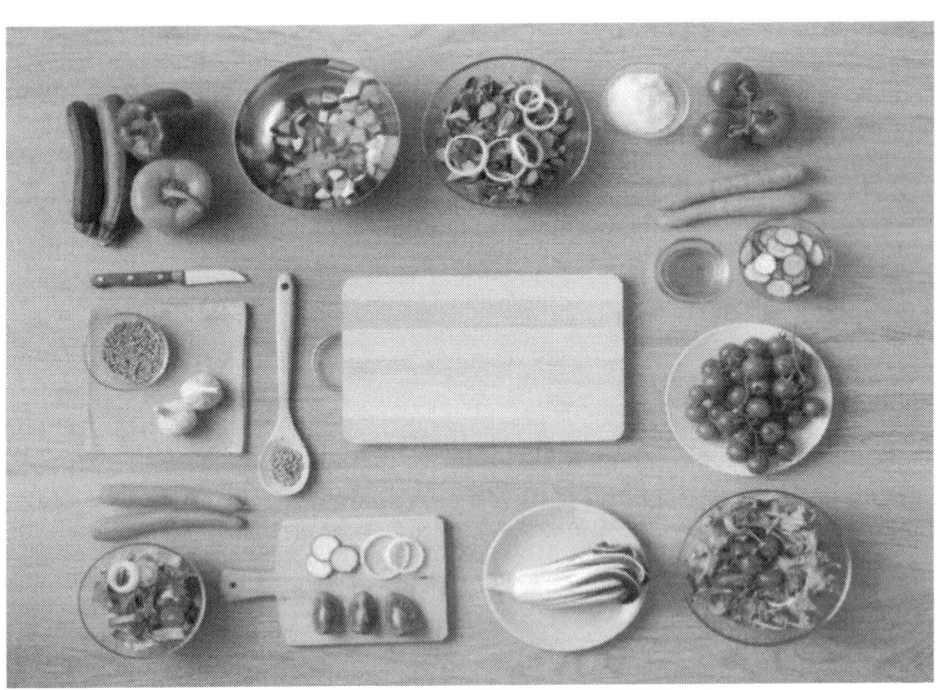

What Is A Vegetarian Ketogenic Diet?

A ketogenic diet is primarily a form of diet wherein the carb intake is restricted to ensure that the body enters a state of ketosis. The energy which is broken down is used for carrying out the different body activities.

In a normal diet in which carbs are regularly consumed, the body is in a state of glycolysis, a process by which carbohydrates are broken down into glucose molecules which are used as energy. However, when the body enters a state of ketosis, as discussed above, fat molecules are used as energy, helping to rid the body of excess fat ensuring weight loss.

Now, shifting our focus to the vegetarian ketogenic diet, the key difference here is that the recipes which we will share will all be vegetarian-based and won't include any kind of meat products whatsoever. The vegetarian ketogenic diet can be followed by both vegetarians and non-vegetarians. So, let us discuss some more details about the vegetarian ketogenic diet.

The Advantages of the Vegetarian Keto Diet Over Other Diets

When compared to most other diets, the vegetarian keto diet surely has many advantages to offer. Let us see the primary ones.

Systematic weight loss: This method of dieting leads to a systematic loss of weight. Do not expect to lose 10 kg in 10 days, but you will see your weight shedding systematically, and you are not likely to put it back again.

Muscular strength: Many forms of dieting are known to lead to loss of muscles as well. When you choose to opt for veg ketogenic diet, you will find that your muscular mass will be retained. You won't become lanky or feel lethargic because your muscles will still have the same kind of strength despite dieting.

You remain vegetarian: One of the best possible things about this diet is that for vegetarians, you do not have to alter your way of living. You still get your vegetarian options and still get to cut down your unwanted pounds without any trouble.

So, with these many possible advantages, it is definitely a recommended form of diet. Now that you have the incentives to opt for this diet form, let us explore more details.

The Aspects of Vegetarian Ketogenic Diet

Let us see some of the core aspects pertaining to this form of ketogenic diet.

The tips First off, a word to the wise: prepare yourself for the keto flu. Many begin the dieting regiment with a great deal of excitement and enthusiasm, but within a week or two, it is likely that some not-so-exciting symptoms will develop. You may feel lethargic, have a mild headache, suffer from nausea, and even lose your appetite for anything and everything. This is what is known as the keto flu, and it is a common reaction your body undergoes when switching from carbs to fat as a source of energy. Stay strong and beat the flu and once the symptoms subside, you will be all set to follow the diet regiment again.

Be mindful of what you are eating. The ketogenic diet mainly aims at cutting down carb intake, but this doesn't mean that you can binge on fat products. You need to be sensible about what you are eating and be logical in your dieting pattern.

Follow the diet regiment thoroughly. It can be a little hard at the beginning, but with time, you should be able to follow it. So, despite the inevitable craving for carbs and high-fat foods, you should try to stay strong and curb the appetite for it. The results will help you in the long run.

The Incentives

Reduces the chance of heart disease

To give you even more incentive for the vegetarian ketogenic diet, let us give you a snapshot of the numerous benefits which you can reap simply from following this dieting pattern.

The keto diet has the potential to reduce the chances of heart disease. While this diet is known to lower the level of bad cholesterol in the body, it also improves the level of good cholesterol. Similarly, the diet can also cut down the level of triglycerides. So, all these cumulative changes are known to help in reducing the chances of heart disease.

Stabilizes the body's metabolism

The keto diet is also known to stabilize the metabolism of the body. While you might experience some taxing side-effects initially, your body will quickly adapt, and it won't be long before you inevitably begin to notice the benefits. Over time, your appetite will be molded by the keto diet regiment, and your body will naturally enter a state of metabolic stability.

Improved energy

The ketogenic diet is also known to result in an increase in energy levels as well. It is very common for people to feel much more energetic and to experience a significant improvement in their ability to focus. So, those who would like to increase their attention span should definitely consider following a vegetarian keto diet.

The Mistakes to Avoid

Now, let us see some of the common mistakes which you should try to avoid.

Do not give up.

No matter how hard it feels initially, stay committed to following the diet. After a week, your body will adjust to the new pattern, and this will help you follow the diet in a much easier way. So, you need to be committed to following the diet.

Do not binge eat.

The ketogenic diet doesn't mean that you can consume as much food as you want as long as it's not carbs. You need to understand the calories you are consuming and be systematic in your diet intake. Avoid carbs and also avoid all kinds of junk food as well.

Stay strong during the keto flu.

Be prepared to be hit by the keto flu and stay strong because this will give you a great head start in following the ketogenic diet. So even when the body feels a little down, stick to your diet, and the flu symptoms are likely to subside in a week or two.

Take care of your health.

Along with the keto diet, you should be mindful of your health. Try and add at least some minor workouts to your routine, such as a short jog, and it should help you stay fit much more easily.

Use these pointers and the positive changes will be apparent.

The Nutrients

Whenever you follow a ketogenic diet, it is important to be mindful of the nutrients. This means you should have an accurate picture of what to eat and what to avoid.

The food to restrict in the ketogenic vegetarian diet

Let us now give you details regarding which food you should exclude from your diet when choosing the vegetarian keto style of eating.

- All grains (even whole grain products) such as oats, barley, sorghum, and rice have to be avoided at all costs.

- You should also avoid things like sugar, honey, maple syrup, and agave as well.

- It's common knowledge that fruit is generally a healthy food choice, but following the keto vegetarian diet means that you need to steer clear of fruits like apple, oranges, and even bananas.

- Lentils, peas, and even black beans should also be avoided.

- Potatoes, yams, and related tubers are on the do-not-eat list as well.

The food to include in the keto vegetarian diet

Now, let us focus on the different foods you are allowed to eat while following this diet.

- Leafy green vegetables, like spinach and kale, are a good choice.

- Vegetables that are grown above ground, like cauliflower, zucchini, and even broccoli, are good options.

- Tempeh, seitan tofu, and any high-protein, low-carb food products are a great addition to a meal.

- Try to include nuts and seeds in your diet. Pumpkin seeds, sunflower seeds, almonds, and pistachios are just a few flavorful options.

- If you're feeling adventurous, try to cook with sea vegetables, such as bladderwrack or kelp.

- Feel free to add fermented foods, like sauerkraut and kimchi, to your meals.

- Foods which have a low glycemic index, including avocado, blackberries, and raspberries, can serve as a nutritious and flavorful addition to your keto vegetarian diet.

So, these are some of the elementary details regarding the ketogenic diet. With these many details, you should now have a very clear picture pertaining to how this whole diet works.

Many people have been following the keto diet for decades now, and there is no mistake that the results are clear and easy to witness. They not only managed to get rid of the extra pounds, but at the same time, they have greatly improved their overall health.

One of the key things which you need to remember when following the veg ketogenic diet is to be the fact that you must follow a systematic and disciplined approach. Your inability to do so would surely hamper the benefits that you would otherwise reap from this diet.

While you have many of the details now, you must be wondering about the possible meals you can cook. We do know that following a strictly vegetarian diet cuts down on many options, and this is why we are going to give you precise recipes which you can follow when making your own meals. With these meals, you will be able to successfully follow the ketogenic diet and observe the changes in your body as well.

How to Get Started

In order to lose weight, you must aim and maintain a calorie deficit. This means burning more energy than you consume. A typical female will consume around 1700 calories daily when dieting, and for men this figure will be roughly 2200, though the ideal target of course differs according to an individual's height, weight, and activity level.

Consuming less than this would be irresponsible. The effects of consuming too few calories can wreak havoc on your body. When you suddenly start consuming much less than your body is used to, it can kick into "starvation mode" and start breaking down muscle instead of fat in an effort to ensure the body's needs are met. This muscle loss will also show up as weight loss on the scale, but it goes without saying that this is not the goal you are attempting to achieve. Avoid retaining your excess fat and lose muscle.

Below are some guidelines to help ensure you are not consuming too many calories for the keto-vegan diet:

Be sure to combat cravings by taking advantage of the satiating effects of protein.

Avoid making the mistake of snacking on too many nuts, seeds, and other fat-rich nibbles when trying to lose weight. These foods are very calorie-dense.

If you have not seen any clear weight loss results after 2-3 weeks, you should consider monitoring your calorie intake closely.

Enjoy the many non-starchy vegetables such as cauliflower, spinach, kale, broccoli, zucchini, and bell peppers, as well as fruits like avocados or berries. These contain many micronutrients in addition to being low in carbs.

Drink water throughout the day the hydrate the body and fill the stomach.

There are two ways you can get started with a keto vegan diet. The first way is by simply jumping right in and cutting out all carbohydrates from your diet. This method can be quite shocking as the transition is very steep. However, the practitioner usually sees results in a quicker time frame and is less likely to deal with sugar withdrawal symptoms for a long period of time.

The second way involves slowly implementing keto vegan practices. This involves slowly reducing your carbohydrate consumption by progressively eating low amounts of carbs every day. The second way is less jarring to beginner practitioners and allows for a learning curve that is not so steep. While it can be easier for newbie keto vegan practitioners to follow the second method, it takes longer to see noticeable results.

The method that you choose to start the keto vegan diet is entirely up to you and depends on your goals and lifestyle. You can start by practicing one method, and then the other to see what works best for you.

No matter how you get started here are a few tips that are useful:

Clear the non-keto vegan foods out of your cupboards and refrigerator and fill them up with keto-vegan friendly food so that you have an easier time sticking to this diet.

Keep things simple at the beginning. Simply up your fat and protein intake and ensure that you are consuming less than 50 grams of carbohydrates every day without worrying too much about the comparative proportions of each. Adjust to the diet then worry about these later.

Consult a licensed health care practitioner before you begin the keto vegan diet. Ensure that you do not have any preexisting medical conditions that might need addressing before you begin this diet.

Foods to Eat

Vegetables

Vegetables contain essential fiber, vitamins, minerals, and phytochemicals. Therefore, it has a high priority in a healthy diet and is vital for our digestive system.

Allowed vegetables:

Spinach, cucumber, broccoli, cauliflower, zucchini, Brussels sprouts, Chinese cabbage, fennel, kale, celeriac, radishes, asparagus, savoy cabbage, asparagus, avocado, bitter green, bok choi, cauliflower, cabbage, celery, chard, cabbage, endive, kohlrabi, lettuce, Nori, olives, radishes, summer squash, artichoke.

Recommendation: In a ketogenic diet, you should focus on low-starch vegetables. However, there is nothing wrong with eating sweet potato, pumpkin, or beetroot now and then.

Healthy fat

Healthy fat is the primary source of energy in a ketogenic diet. Approximately 70-80% of all calories should come from this category.

Allowed fat:

Coconut oil, olive oil, avocado oil, MCT oil, caprylic acid, krill oil, vegan butter, grape ghee, sunflower lecithin, almond paste, cocoa butter.

Recommendation: Consume at least two tablespoons of MCT oil or pure caprylic acid daily. The body converts the medium-chain fatty acids contained into three metabolic steps.

High-quality proteins

For a properly conducted ketogenic diet, one should not exaggerate the protein consumption.

Allowed foods:

Grape-based collagen hydrolysate, vegetable protein powder.

Recommendation: Do not overdo protein consumption. Instead, pay good attention to the quality of your protein source.

Fruits and berries

Although fruits contain vitamins and minerals, they often also contain large amounts of fructose. You can measure the effect on your ketosis.

Allowed:

Blueberries, strawberries, blackberries, raspberries, elderberries, currants, avocado, papaya.

Recommendation: Focus on low-sugar fruits such as berries. Treat her like some sweets. For example, you can make a delicious berry sorbet with frozen blueberries for dessert.

Drinks

Water, water with lemon juice, herbal tea, coffee, high-quality green tea, homemade lemonade, homemade ice tea, coconut milk, and almond milk (unsweetened).

Recommendation: It is essential to drink enough water. Try to take at least 2-3 liters of fluid daily.

Nuts and seeds

Macadamia, almond, coconut, pecans, walnuts, and cashews.

Recommendation: Since nuts are rich in trace elements, but also contain anti-nutrients such as phytic acid, you should limit the consumption to a handful per day.

Ketogenic alternatives

Keto Mayonnaise, Keto Biscuits, 85% Chocolate, Keto Cocoa, Keto Energy Balls, Keto Gummy Bears.

Recommendation: It is always practical to have delicious and ketogenic alternatives to the small sins of the diet at home. For example, in our office, we always have ketogenic mayonnaise and ketogenic biscuits.

Foods to Avoid

Of course, you should be careful to keep your consumption of carbohydrates low in a ketogenic diet. But by now, you have also learned that we are not only concerned with the macronutrients, but also the quality of the food to eat and the effect on your health.

Here you can find out which foods are not part of a healthy ketogenic diet.

Sugar in all forms

Sugar (sucrose), corn syrup (GFS, HFCS), agave syrup, molasses, brown sugar, granulated sugar, cane sugar, caramel, coconut sugar, palm sugar, sugarcane juice, fruit juice, fruit juice concentrate, sugar beet syrup, glucose, invert sugar, molasses.

Ketogenic alternative: xylitol, erythritol, stevia, ribose, primal sweet.

Artificial additives / food

Artificial flavors, artificial colors, artificial sugar substitutes, trans fat, bouillon.

Ketogenic alternative: real ingredients that provide real flavors!

Cereal products

Cereal products contain large amounts of fast carbohydrates and will immediately kick you out of ketosis. Therefore, you should avoid them. This includes:

Bread, pasta, cake, biscuits, pizza, cornmeal

Tip: You do not have to do without tasty pasta entirely if you know the right alternatives. For example, there is super delicious gluten-free bread or ketogenic spaghetti.

Alternatives: coconut flour, almond flour.

A Meal Plan for your First Month

Day	Breakfast	Lunch	Snack	Dinner	Dessert
1	Coconut Porridge with Blackberries	Delish Carrots	Nori Snack Rolls	Seitan Tex-Mex Casserole	Strawberry Coconut Parfait
2	Strawberry Chia Pudding	Glazed Carrots	Risotto Bites	Avocado Coconut Pie	Lemon-Chocolate Truffles
3	Raspberry Almond Smoothie	Sweet & Spicy Carrots	Jicama and Guacamole	Baked Mushrooms with Creamy Brussels Sprouts	Blackberry and Red Wine Crumble
4	Vanilla Yogurt Pancakes	Bell Pepper Gumbo	Curried Tofu "Egg Salad" Pitas	Pimiento Tofu balls	Cinnamon-Chocolate Cake
5	Broccoli Hash Browns	Italian Bell Pepper Platter	Garden Patch Sandwiches on Multigrain Bread	Tempeh with Garlic Asparagus	Himalayan Raspberry Fat Bombs
6	Sesame-Chia Bread	Green Goddess Buddha Bowl	Garden Salad Wraps	Mushroom Curry Pie	Cashew-Chocolate Cheesecake
7	No-Bread Avocado Sandwich	Cauliflower Rice and Mushroom Risotto	Black Sesame Wonton Chips	Spicy Cheese with Tofu Balls	Creamy Avocado Drink
8	Pear Oatmeal	Grilled Eggplant Roll-Ups	Marinated Mushroom Wraps	Tempeh Coconut Curry Bake	Raspberry Cookies
9	Pumpkin Oatmeal	Eggplant Gratin with Feta Cheese	Tamari Toasted Almonds	Kale and Mushroom Pierogis	Lenny & Larry's Cookies

10	Veggie Burrito	Tofu Pesto Zoodles	Avocado and Tempeh Bacon Wraps	Mushroom Lettuce Wraps	Zucchini Chocolate Brownies
11	Apple Steel Cut Oats	Cheesy Mushroom Pie	Kale Chips	Tofu and Spinach Lasagna with Red Sauce	Fudgy Pumpkin Brownies
12	Tofu Casserole	Meatless Florentine Pizza	Tempeh-Pimiento Cheese Ball	Green Avocado Carbonara	Cinnamon Roll Bars
13	Carrot Mix	Margherita Pizza with Cauliflower Crust	Seaweed Crackers	Cashew Buttered Quesadillas with Leafy Greens	Snickers Bars
14	Blueberries Oats	Almond Tofu Loaf	Sesame Tamari Almonds	Zucchini Boats with Vegan Cheese	Lemon Coconut Crack Bars
15	Apple and Pears Mix	Kale and Mushroom Biryani	Edamame Avocado Hummus	Tempeh Garam Masala Bake	Gingerbread Cookie Bars
16	Bell Pepper Oatmeal	Mushroom Pizza Bowls with Avocado & Cilantro	Pizza Cheese Ball	Caprese Casserole	Cocoa Berries Mousse
17	Banana and Walnuts Oats	Pistachios and Cheese Stuffed Zucchinis	Tahini Keto Bagels	Lemon Garlic Mushrooms	Nutmeg Pudding
18	Simple Granola	Soy Chorizo-Asparagus Bowl	Zucchini Nests	Almond Green Beans	Lime Cherries and Rice Pudding
19	Zucchini Oatmeal	Creamy Brussels Sprouts Bowls	Low Carb Bibimbap	Fried Okra	Chocolate Pudding
20	Cranberry Coconut Quinoa	Green Beans and Radishes Bake	Walnut Carrot Bombs	Super Healthy Beet Greens Salad	Coffee and Rhubarb Cream

21	Gingerbread Porridge	Avocado and Radish Bowls	Nutty Zucchini Salad	Coconut Yogurt with Chia Seeds and Almonds	Chocolate Sea Salt Almonds
22	Overnight Strawberry Cheesecake Porridge	Celery and Radish Soup	Kale Pate Spread	Super Delicious Cucumber Salad	Salted Caramel Cashew Brittle
23	Blueberry Quinoa Porridge	Lime Avocado and Cucumber Soup	Smoked Almonds	Pudding Delight with Banana & Coconut	Cookies and Cream Parfait
24	Blueberry Chia Pudding	Avocado and Kale Soup	Roasted Garlic Mushrooms	Extra Easy Cheese Sandwich	Pecan Pie Pudding
25	Almond Flour Muffins	Spinach and Cucumber Salad	Mediterranean Cucumber Bites	India Super Easy Summer Cooler	Chocolate Avocado Pudding
26	Coconut Porridge with Blackberries	Delish Carrots	Nori Snack Rolls	Seitan Tex-Mex Casserole	Strawberry Coconut Parfait
27	Strawberry Chia Pudding	Glazed Carrots	Risotto Bites	Avocado Coconut Pie	Lemon-Chocolate Truffles
28	Raspberry Almond Smoothie	Sweet & Spicy Carrots	Jicama and Guacamole	Baked Mushrooms with Creamy Brussels Sprouts	Blackberry and Red Wine Crumble
29	Vanilla Yogurt Pancakes	Bell Pepper Gumbo	Curried Tofu "Egg Salad" Pitas	Pimiento Tofu balls	Cinnamon-Chocolate Cake
30	Broccoli Hash Browns	Italian Bell Pepper Platter	Garden Patch Sandwiches on Multigrain Bread	Tempeh with Garlic Asparagus	Himalayan Raspberry Fat Bombs

Breakfast Recipes

1. Coconut Porridge with Blackberries

Preparation Time: 7 Minutes

Cooking Time: 5 Minutes

Servings: 4

Ingredients:

For the flax egg:

1 tbsp flax seed powder + 3 tbsp water

1 tbsp olive oil

1 tbsp coconut flour

1 pinch ground chia seeds

5 tbsp coconut cream

1 pinch salt

Thawed frozen blackberries to serve

Directions:

In a small bowl, mix the flax seed powder with the water and allow thickening for 5 minutes.

Place a non-stick saucepan over low heat and mix all the ingredients except for the blackberries. Cook the mixture while stirring continuously until your desired thickness is achieved.

Turn the heat off and spoon the porridge into serving bowls.

Top with some blackberries and serve immediately.

Nutrition:

Calories:131 Cal Fat:13.3 g

Carbs: 3 g Fiber: 1g Protein:2 g

2. Strawberry Chia Pudding

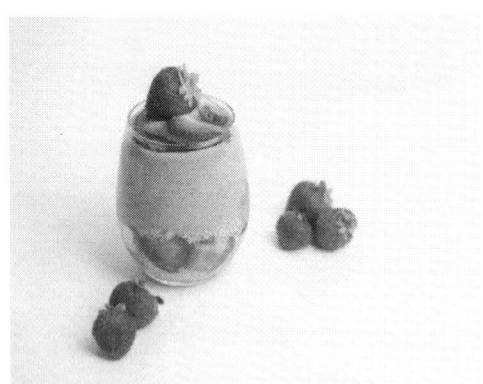

Preparation Time: 10 Minutes

Cooking Time: 0

Servings: 4

Ingredients:

1 ½ cups coconut milk

½ cup dairy-free plain yogurt

4 tsp sugar-free maple syrup

1 tsp vanilla extract

7 tbsp chia seeds

1 cup fresh strawberries + extra for garnishing

Chopped almonds to garnish

Mint leaves to garnish

Directions:

In a bowl, mix all the ingredients up to the chia seeds.

Mash the strawberries in a bowl using a fork and stir the puree into the yogurt mixture.

Divide the mix into four medium mason jars, cover the lids and refrigerate for 30 minutes to thicken the pudding.

Take out the jars, remove the lids, and stir the pudding. Garnish with two strawberries each, almonds, and some mint leaves.

Serve immediately.

Nutrition:

Calories: 240 Cal

Fat:22.6 g

Carbs: 9 g

Fiber: 3 g

Pro tein: 3 g

3. Raspberry Almond Smoothie

Preparation Time: 2 Minutes

Cooking Time: 0

Servings: 4

Ingredients:

1 ½ cups almond milk or coconut milk

3 tbsp coconut cream

½ cup raspberries

Juice from half lemon

½ tsp almond extract

Directions:

Process all the ingredients in a high-speed blender until smooth.

Pour into serving cups and enjoy.

Nutrition:

Calories:216 Cal

Fat:21.7 g

Carbs: 7 g

Fiber: 3g

Protein:3 g

4. Vanilla Yogurt Pancakes

Preparation Time: 8 Minutes

Cooking Time: 15 Minutes

Servings: 4

Ingredients:

½ cup almond flour

½ tsp baking powder

1 tbsp erythritol

½ cup dairy-free plain yogurt

1 lemon, juiced

1 vanilla pod, caviar extracted

2 tbsp unsalted vegan butter

2 tbsp olive oil

Sugar-free maple syrup to serve

Dairy-free plain yogurt to serve

Choice of berries to serve

Directions:

Sift the almond flour and baking powder into a medium bowl and mix in the erythritol.

In a small bowl, whisk the yogurt, lemon juice. Combine both mixtures, add the vanilla caviar and whisk well until smooth.

In a medium skillet set over medium heat, melt a quarter each of the vegan butter and olive oil. Add 1 ½ tablespoons of the pancake mixture into the pan and cook for 3 to 4 minutes or until small bubbles begin to show.

Flip the pancake and cook the other side until set and golden, 2 minutes. Repeat cooking until the batter finishes using the remaining vegan butter and olive oil in the same proportions.

Plate the pancakes, drizzle with some maple syrup, top with a generous dollop of yogurt, and scatter some berries on top.

Serve immediately.

Nutrition:

Calories:165 Cal

Fat: 14.9g

Carbs: 3 g,

Fiber:0 g

Protein:6 g

5. Broccoli Hash Browns

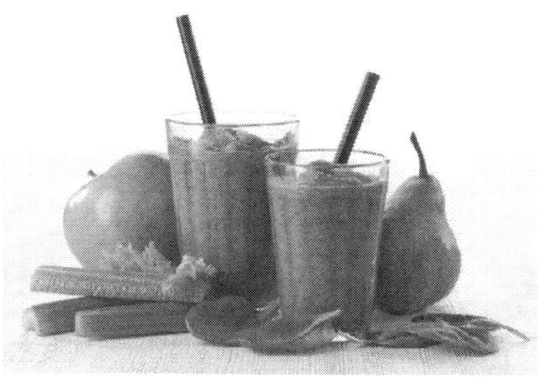

Preparation Time: 10 Minutes

Cooking Time: 24 Minutes

Servings: 4

Ingredients:

3 tbsp flax seed powder + 9 tbsp water

1 big head broccoli, riced

½ white onion, grated

1 tsp salt

1 tbsp black pepper

5 tbsp vegan butter, for frying

Directions:

In a medium bowl, mix the flax seed powder with the water and allow thickening for 5 minutes.

Mix in the broccoli, onion, salt, and black pepper. Allow sitting for 5 minutes to thicken the mixture.

Place a large non-stick skillet over medium heat and melt in 1/3 of the vegan butter.

Ladle scoops of the broccoli mixture into the skillet (about 3 to 4 hash browns per batch), flatten the pancakes to measure 3 to 4 inches in diameter and fry until golden brown on one side, 4 minutes.

Turn the pancakes and cook the other side until brown too, 5 minutes.

Plate the pancakes, make more, and serve warm.

Nutrition:

Calories: 216 Cal Fat:21.3 g

Carbs:5 g Fiber:2 g, Protein:4 g

6. Sesame-Chia Bread

Preparation Time: 10minutes

Cooking Time: 45minutes

Servings: 6

Ingredients:

3 tbsp ground flax seeds

½ cup + 1 tbsp water

2/3 cup cream cheese, room temperature

¼ cup melted coconut oil

2 tbsp sesame oil

¾ cup coconut cream

¾ cup coconut flour

1 cup almond flour

3 tsp baking powder

5 1/3 tbsp sesame seeds

½ cup chia seeds

¼ cup psyllium husk powder

1 tsp salt   1 tbsp poppy seeds

Directions:

Preheat the oven to 350 F and line a 4 x 7-inch loaf pan with baking paper.

In a medium bowl, whisk the flax seed powder with the water, and allow soaking for 5 minutes.

Using an electric hand mixer, whisk in the cream cheese, coconut oil, sesame oil, and coconut cream.

In another bowl, mix the coconut flour, almond flour, baking powder, sesame seeds, chia seeds, psyllium husk powder, and salt.

Blend both mixtures until dough forms.

Transfer the dough to the loaf pan, sprinkle with the poppy seeds, and bake in the oven for 45 minutes or until a skewer inserted into the bread comes out clean.

Remove the parchment paper with the bread and allow cooling on a rack.

Slice and serve the bread for breakfast.

Nutrition: Calories: 570 Fat: 57.6g

Carbs: 12 g Fiber:5 g Protein:10 g

7. No-Bread Avocado Sandwich

Preparation Time: 10 Minutes

Cooking Time: 0

Servings: 2

Ingredients:

2 oz. little gem lettuce, 2 leaves extracted

½ oz vegan butter

1 oz sliced vegan cheese

1 avocado, pitted, peeled, and sliced

1 large red tomato, sliced

Chopped fresh parsley to garnish

Directions:

Rinse and pat dry the lettuce leave. Arrange on a flat plate (with inner side facing you) to serve as the base of the sandwich.

Spread some butter on each leaf, top with the cheese, avocado, and tomato.

Garnish with some parsley and serve the sandwich immediately.

Nutrition:

Calories:143 Cal

Fat: 12.7g

Carbs:6 g

Fiber: 4 g

Protein: 4g

8. Pear Oatmeal

Preparation Time: 10 Minutes

Cooking Time: 15 Minutes

Servings: 3

Ingredients:

2 cups coconut milk

½ cup steel cut oats

½ teaspoon vanilla extract

1 pear, chopped

½ teaspoon maple extract

1 tablespoon stevia

Directions:

In your air fryer's pan, mix coconut milk with oats, vanilla, pear, maple extract and stevia, stir, cover and cook at 360 degrees F for 15 minutes.

Divide into bowls and serve for breakfast.

Enjoy!

Nutrition:

Calories: 200 Cal

Fat: 5 g

Fiber: 7 g

Carbs 14 g

Protein: 4 g

9. Pumpkin Oatmeal

Preparation Time: 10 Minutes

Cooking Time: 20 Minutes

Servings: 4

Ingredients:

1 and ½ cups water

½ cup pumpkin puree

1 teaspoon pumpkin pie spice

3 tablespoons stevia

½ cup steel cut oats

Directions:

In your air fryer's pan, mix water with oats, pumpkin puree, pumpkin spice and stevia, stir, cover and cook at 360 degrees F for 20 minutes

Divide into bowls and serve for breakfast.

Enjoy!

Nutrition:

Calories: 21 Cal

Fat: $ g

Fiber: 7 g

Carbs 8 g

Protein: 3 g

10. Veggie Burrito

Preparation Time: 10 Minutes

Cooking Time: 15 Minutes

Servings: 8

Ingredients:

16 ounces tofu, crumbled

1 green bell pepper, chopped

¼ cup scallions, chopped

15 ounces canned black beans, drained

1 cup vegan salsa

½ cup water

¼ teaspoon cumin, ground

½ teaspoon turmeric powder

½ teaspoon smoked paprika

A pinch of salt and black pepper

¼ teaspoon chili powder

3 cups spinach leaves, torn

8 vegan tortillas for serving

Directions:

In your air fryer, mix tofu with bell pepper, scallions, black beans, salsa, water, cumin, turmeric, paprika, salt, pepper and chili powder, stir, cover and cook at 370 degrees F for 20 minutes

Add spinach, toss well, divide this on your vegan tortillas, roll, wrap them and serve for breakfast.

Enjoy!

Nutrition:

Calories: 211 Cal

Fat: 4 g

Fiber: 7 g

Carbs 14 g

Protein: 4 g

11. Apple Steel Cut Oats

Preparation Time: 10 Minutes

Cooking Time: 15 Minutes

Servings: 6

Ingredients:

1 and ½ cups water

1 and ½ cups coconut milk

2 apples, cored, peeled and chopped

1 cup steel cut oats

½ teaspoon cinnamon powder

¼ teaspoon nutmeg, ground

¼ teaspoon allspice, ground

¼ teaspoon ginger powder

¼ teaspoon cardamom, ground

1 tablespoon flaxseed, ground

2 teaspoons vanilla extract

2 teaspoons stevia

Cooking spray

Directions:

Spray your air fryer with cooking spray, add apples, milk, water, cinnamon, oats, allspice, nutmeg, cardamom, ginger, vanilla, flaxseeds and stevia, stir, cover and cook at 360 degrees F for 15 minutes

Divide into bowls and serve for breakfast.

Enjoy!

Nutrition:

Calories: 172 Cal

Fat: 3 g

Fiber: 7 g

Carbs 8 g

Protein: 5 g

12. Tofu Casserole

Preparation Time: 10 Minutes

Cooking Time: 20 Minutes

Servings: 4

Ingredients:

1 teaspoon lemon zest, grated

14 ounces tofu, cubed

1 tablespoon lemon juice

2 tablespoons nutritional yeast

1 tablespoon apple cider vinegar

1 tablespoon olive oil

2 garlic cloves, minced

10 ounces spinach, torn

½ cup yellow onion, chopped

½ teaspoon basil, dried

8 ounces mushrooms, sliced

Salt and black pepper to the taste

¼ teaspoon red pepper flakes

Cooking spray

Directions:

Spray your air fryer with some cooking spray, arrange tofu cubes on the bottom, add lemon zest, lemon juice, yeast, vinegar, olive oil, garlic, spinach, onion, basil, mushrooms, salt, pepper and pepper flakes, toss, cover and cook at 365 degrees F for 20 minutes.

Divide between plates and serve for breakfast.

Enjoy!

Nutrition Value: calories 246, fat 6, fiber 8, carbs 12, protein 4

Nutrition: Calories: 2460 Cal

Fat: 6 g Fiber: 8 g Carbs 12 g Protein: 4 g

13. Carrot Mix

Preparation Time: 10 Minutes

Cooking Time: 15 Minutes

Servings: 4

Ingredients:

2 cups coconut milk

½ cup steel cut oats

1 cup carrots, shredded

1 teaspoon cardamom, ground

½ teaspoon agave nectar

A pinch of saffron

Cooking spray

Directions:

Spray your air fryer with cooking spray, add milk, oats, carrots, cardamom and agave nectar, stir, cover and cook at 365 degrees F for 15 minutes

Divide into bowls, sprinkle saffron on top and serve for breakfast.

Enjoy!

Nutrition Value: calories 202, fat 7, fiber 4, carbs 8, protein 3

Nutrition:

Calories: 202 Cal Fat: 7 g

Fiber: 4 g Carbs 8 g

Protein: 8 g

14. Blueberries Oats

Preparation Time: 10 Minutes

Cooking Time: 15 Minutes

Servings: 4

Ingredients:

1 cup blueberries

1 cup steel cut oats

1 cup coconut milk

2 tablespoons agave nectar

½ teaspoon vanilla extract

Cooking spray

Directions:

Spray your air fryer with cooking spray, add oats, milk, agave nectar, vanilla and blueberries, toss, cover and cook at 365 degrees F for 10 minutes.

Divide into bowls and serve for breakfast.

Enjoy!

Nutrition:

Calories: 202 Cal

Fat: 6 g

Fiber: 8 g

Carbs 9g

Protein: 6 g

15. Apple and Pears Mix

Preparation Time: 10 Minutes

Cooking Time: 15 Minutes

Servings: 6

Ingredients:

4 apples, cored, peeled and cut into medium chunks

1 teaspoon lemon juice

4 pears, cored, peeled and cut into medium chunks

5 teaspoons stevia

1 teaspoon cinnamon powder

1 teaspoon vanilla extract

½ teaspoon ginger, ground

½ teaspoon cloves, ground

½ teaspoon cardamom, ground

Directions:

In your air fryer, mix apples with pears, lemon juice, stevia, cinnamon, vanilla extract, ginger, cloves and cardamom, stir, cover, cook at 360 degrees F for 15 minutes

Divide into bowls and serve for breakfast.

Enjoy!

Nutrition:

Calories:161 Cal

Fat: 3 g Fiber: 7 g Carbs 9 g Protein: 4 g

16. Bell Pepper Oatmeal

Preparation Time: 10 Minutes

Cooking Time: 15 Minutes

Servings: 2

Ingredients:

1 cup steel cut oats

2 tablespoons canned kidney beans, drained

2 red bell peppers, chopped

4 tablespoons coconut cream

A pinch of sweet paprika

Salt and black pepper to the taste

¼ teaspoon cumin, ground

Directions:

Heat up your air fryer at 360 degrees F, add oats, beans, bell peppers, coconut cream, paprika, salt, pepper and cumin, stir, cover and cook for 16 minutes.

Divide into bowls and serve for breakfast.

Enjoy!

Nutrition:

Calories: 173Cal

Fat: 4 g Fiber: 6 g

Carbs 12 g Protein: 4 g

17. Banana and Walnuts Oats

Preparation Time: 10 Minutes

Cooking Time: 15 Minutes

Servings: 4

Ingredients:

1 banana, peeled and mashed

1 cup steel cut oats

2 cups almond milk

2 cups water

¼ cup walnuts, chopped

2 tablespoons flaxseed meal

2 teaspoons cinnamon powder

1 teaspoon vanilla extract

½ teaspoon nutmeg, ground

Directions:

In your air fryer mix oats with almond milk, water, walnuts, flaxseed meal, cinnamon, vanilla and nutmeg, stir, cover and cook at 360 degrees F for 15 minutes.

Divide into bowls and serve for breakfast.

Enjoy!

Nutrition:

Calories: 181 Cal

Fat: 7 g Fiber: 6 g Carbs 12 g

Protein: 11 g

18. Simple Granola

Preparation Time: 10 Minutes

Cooking Time: 15 Minutes

Servings: 3

Ingredients:

½ cup granola

½ cup bran flakes

2 green apples, cored, peeled and roughly chopped

¼ cup apple juice

1/8 cup maple syrup

2 tablespoons cashew butter

1 teaspoon cinnamon powder

½ teaspoon nutmeg, ground

Directions:

In your air fryer, mix granola with bran flakes, apples, apple juice, maple syrup, cashew butter, cinnamon and nutmeg, toss, cover and cook at 365 degrees F for 15 minutes

Divide into bowls and serve for breakfast.

Enjoy!

Nutrition:

Calories: 188 Cal

Fat: 6 g Fiber: 9 g

Carbs 11 g Protein: 6 g

19. Zucchini Oatmeal

Preparation Time: 10 Minutes

Cooking Time: 15 Minutes

Servings: 4

Ingredients:

½ cup steel cut oats

1 carrot, grated

1 and ½ cups almond milk

¼ zucchini, grated

¼ teaspoon nutmeg, ground

¼ teaspoon cloves, ground

½ teaspoon cinnamon powder

2 tablespoons maple syrup

¼ cup pecans, chopped

1 teaspoon vanilla extract

Directions:

In your air fryer, mix oats with carrot, zucchini, almond milk, cloves, nutmeg, cinnamon, maple syrup, pecans and vanilla extract, stir, cover and cook at 365 degrees F for 15 minutes.

Divide into bowls and serve.

Enjoy!

Nutrition:

Calories: 175 Cal Fat: 4 g

Fiber: 7 g Carbs 12 g Protein: 7 g

20. Cranberry Coconut Quinoa

Preparation Time: 10 Minutes

Cooking Time: 13 Minutes

Servings: 4

Ingredients:

1 cup quinoa

3 cups coconut water

1 teaspoon vanilla extract

3 teaspoons stevia

1/8 cup coconut flakes

¼ cup cranberries, dried

1/8 cup almonds, chopped

Directions:

In your air fryer, mix quinoa with coconut water, vanilla, stevia, coconut flakes, almonds and cranberries, toss, cover and cook at 365 degrees F for 13 minutes.

Divide into bowls and serve for breakfast.

Enjoy!

Nutrition:

Calories: 146 Cal

Fat: 5 g

Fiber: 5 g

Carbs 10 g Protein: 7 g

21. Gingerbread Porridge

Preparation Time: 9 Minutes

Cooking Time: 2 Minutes

Servings: 2

Ingredients:

1/3 c. coconut milk, full-fat, canned

½ c. water

1 tbsp. coconut flour

¼ c. hemp seeds

½ c. flacked unsweetened coconut

1 ½ t. ground ginger

1 t. of the following:

ground cloves

ground nutmeg

vanilla

½ tbsp. ground cinnamon

1-2 teaspoons sweetener of your choice

Optional Toppings

Almond butter, chopped walnuts/pecans, cranberries

Directions:

In a medium saucepan, add the milk, water, coconut, coconut flour, & hemp seed.

Bring these ingredients to a boil, allowing to simmer 2 minutes or until thickened.

Add cinnamon, vanilla ginger, cloves, nutmeg, and combine until well-mixed and put in a heat-resistant bowl.

Sprinkle sweetener and any optional toppings of your choice across the top.

Mix and enjoy with additional milk as needed.

Nutrition:

Calories: 374 Cal

Proteins: 11 g

Carbos: 9 g

Fats: 33 g

22. Overnight Strawberry Cheesecake Porridge

Preparation Time: 10 Minutes

Cooking Time: 0

Servings: 1

Ingredients

¼ c. fresh strawberries

½ c. coconut milk

2 tbsp. of the following:

coconut yogurt

ground flaxseed

chia seeds

sweetener of your choice

1 tbsp. of the following:

almond flour

shredded unsweetened coconut

Directions:

Mix almond flour, unsweetened coconut, sweetener, chia seed, and flaxseed in a shallow bowl.

Next, pour ¼ cup of the coconut milk with dry contents and combine well.

Refrigerate overnight.

Before serving, add the remaining milk until the mixture becomes thick and creamy.

Layer the yogurt and strawberries on top.

Mix and enjoy.

Nutrition:

Calories: 275 Cal

Proteins: 8 g

Carbs: 16 g

Fats: 17 g

23. Blueberry Quinoa Porridge

Preparation Time: 20 Minutes

Cooking Time: 15 Minutes

Servings: 2

Ingredients:

1 c. blueberries

1/8 t. cinnamon

¼ t. vanilla

1 tbsp. sweetener of your choice

2 c. almond milk

1 c. uncooked quinoa

Optional Toppings

Chia seeds, hemp seeds, hazelnuts

Directions:

In a saucepan, add milk and quinoa.

Heat milk and quinoa at low heat for roughly 10 minutes, stirring to prevent scorching.

Slowly combine vanilla, cinnamon, and sugar and cook for 5 minutes or when the quinoa soft.

Take away from the heat and place in serving bowls.

Top with blueberries and sprinkle sweetener of your choice across the top.

Mix and enjoy.

Nutrition:

Calories: 374 Cal

Proteins: 11 g

Carbs: 9 g

Fats: 33 g

24. Blueberry Chia Pudding

Preparation Time: 8 Hours 10 Minutes

Cooking Time: 0

Servings: 3

Ingredients

1/8 t. cinnamon

½ t. vanilla

2 c. almond milk, unsweetened

1 tbsp. maple syrup

1/3 c. blueberries

6 tbsp. chia seeds, fresh

Directions:

Combine the chia seeds, blueberries, syrup, milk, vanilla, and cinnamon into a blender, blending into a silky consistency.

Separate mixture into 3 glasses or ramekins.

Chill overnight or until set, approximately 8 hours.

Enjoy it chilled.

Nutrition:

Calories: 374

Proteins: 11 g

Cars: 9 g

Fats: 33 g

25. Almond Flour Muffins

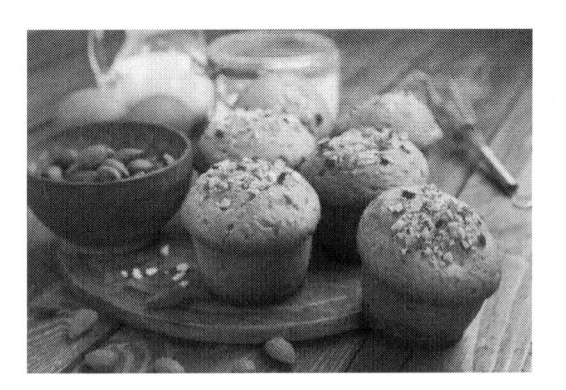

Preparation Time: 10 Minutes

Cooking Time: 15 Minutes

Servings: 4

Ingredients

¼ t. salt

½ tbsp. baking powder

1 flax egg

¼ c. almond milk

1 tbsp. stevia (or your sweetener of choice)

1 c. almond flour

Olive oil for greasing muffin pan.

Optional add-in

Crushed, walnuts, blueberries, sugar-free chocolate chips

Directions:

Set the oven to preheat at 35

Grease the muffin pan with olive oil.

Combine baking powder, stevia, salt, and almond flour in a mixing bowl. Mix completely.

Slowly add the flax egg and almond milk and mix well

If adding any add-ins, add them at this point (crushed walnuts, blueberries, chocolate chips).

Using a ¼ c. measuring cup, fill each muffin tin approximately 2/3 full.

Carefully slide into the oven and cook for 10 minutes (mini size) or 15 minutes (regular size).

Take it from oven and place in a cool area to allow muffins to cool while still in the tin for about 10 minutes. Then, carefully remove the muffins using a knife to loosen them from the sides of the tin.

Nutrition:

Calories: 217 Cal

Proteins: 11 g

Carbs: 9 g

Fats: 33 g

Lunch Recipes

26. Delish Carrots

Preparation Time: 15 Minutes

Cooking Time: 20 Minutes

Servings: 16

Ingredients:

2 tbsp. olive oil

1 chopped yellow onion

3 finely chopped garlic cloves

5 pounds halved medium baby carrots baby

½ cup homemade vegetable broth

1 tsp Italian seasoning

1 tsp spike seasoning

Directions:

Place the oil in the Instant Pot and select "Sauté". Then add the onion and garlic and cook for about 4-5 minutes.

Add the carrots and cook for about 4-5 minutes.

Select the "Cancel" and stir in collard greens and water.

Secure the lid and place the pressure valve to "Seal" position.

Select "Manual" and cook under "High Pressure" for about 10 minutes.

Select the "Cancel" and carefully do a "Natural" release for about 10 minutes and then do a "Quick" release.

Remove the lid and serve.

Nutrition:

Calories: 70 Cal Fat: 2.1g

Carbs: 0.78g Protein: 1.2g Fiber: 4.3g

27. Glazed Carrots

Preparation Time: 15 Minutes

Cooking Time: 4 Minutes

Servings: 8

Ingredients: 2 pounds baby carrots

1/3 cup butter 2 tbsp. Erythritol

1/2 tsp ground cinnamon

salt, to taste ½ cup water

Directions:

In the pot of Instant Pot, add all ingredients and stir to combine.

Secure the lid and place the pressure valve to "Seal" position.

Select "Manual" and cook under "High Pressure" for about 4 minutes.

Select the "Cancel" and carefully do a "Natural" release.

Remove the lid and serve.

Nutrition:

Calories: 91 Fat: 5.9g Carbs: 1.56g

Protein: 0.8g Fiber: 3.4g

28. Sweet & Spicy Carrots

Preparation Time: 18 Minutes

Cooking Time: 2 Minutes

Servings: 4

Ingredients:

1 pound quartered lengthwise and halved carrots

1 tbsp. Erythritol

2 tbsp. butter

3 tsp ground mustard

1 tsp ground cumin

½ tsp cayenne pepper

¼ tsp red pepper flakes

Salt and freshly ground black pepper, to taste

1/8 tsp ground cinnamon

Directions:

In the bottom of Instant Pot, arrange a steamer basket and pour 1 cup of water.

Place the carrots into the steamer basket.

Secure the lid and place the pressure valve to "Seal" position.

Select "Manual" and cook under "High Pressure" for about 1 minute.

Select the "Cancel" and carefully do a "Quick" release.

Remove the lid and transfer the carrots to a bowl.

Remove water from the pot and with paper towels, pat dry.

Select the "Sauté" mode for Power Pressure Cooker. In the pot of Pressure Cooker, melt butter and stir in the remaining ingredients.

Stir in the carrots and cook for about 1 minute.

Select the "Cancel" and serve warm with the sprinkling of cinnamon.

Nutrition:

Calories: 112

Fat: 6.6g Carbs: 3.50g Protein: 1.7g

Fiber: 3.3g

29. Bell Pepper Gumbo

Preparation Time: 20 Minutes

Cooking Time: 5 Minutes

Servings: 3

Ingredients:

tbsp. olive oil

4 minced garlic cloves

½ tsp cumin seeds

1 seeded and cut into long strips green bell pepper

1 seeded and cut into long strips red bell pepper

1 seeded and cut into long strips yellow bell pepper

1 seeded and cut into long strips bell pepper

½ tsp red chili powder

¼ tsp ground turmeric

Salt and freshly ground black pepper, to taste

¼ cup water

½ tbsp. fresh lemon juice

Directions:

Place the oil in the Instant Pot and select "Sauté". Then add the garlic and cumin and cook for about 1 minute.

Select the "Cancel" and stir in remaining ingredients except for lemon juice.

Secure the lid and place the pressure valve to "Seal" position.

Select "Manual" and cook under "High Pressure" for about 2 minutes.

Select the "Cancel" and carefully do a "Quick" release.

Remove the lid and select "Sauté".

Stir in lemon juice and cook for about 1-2 minutes.

Select the "Cancel" and serve.

Nutrition:

Calories 101 Total Fat 5.3g

Net Carbs 4.6g Protein 2g Fiber 2.5g

30. Italian Bell Pepper Platter

Preparation Time: 20 Minutes

Cooking Time: 10 Minutes

Servings: 5

Ingredients: tbsp. olive oil

1 cut into thin strips yellow onion

5 seeded and cut into long strips green bell peppers

very finely chopped medium ripe tomatoes

chopped garlic cloves

tbsp. fresh parsley

Salt and freshly ground black pepper, to taste

Directions:

Place the oil in the Instant Pot and select "Sauté". Then add the onion and cook for about 3-4 minutes.

Add the bell peppers and garlic clove and cook for about 5 minutes.

Select the "Cancel" and stir in remaining ingredients.

Secure the lid and place the pressure valve to "Seal" position.

Select "Manual" and cook under "High Pressure" for about 5-6 minutes.

Select the "Cancel" and carefully do a "Quick" release.

Remove the lid and serve.

Nutrition:

Calories 82 Total Fat 3.2g

Net Carbs 2.7g Protein 12.4g Fiber 2.7g

31. Green Goddess Buddha Bowl

Preparation Time: 10 Minutes

Cooking Time: 5 Minutes

Servings: 1

Ingredients:

2 cups fresh spinach

2 tablespoons avocado oil

4 broccolini spears

⅛ teaspoon salt

⅛ teaspoon freshly ground black pepper

⅓ cup frozen cauliflower rice, thawed

2 tablespoons shredded carrots

½ avocado, sliced

1 tablespoon almond butter, melted

1 tablespoon minced fresh cilantro

Directions:

Place the spinach in the bottom of a medium serving bowl.

In a skillet over medium-high heat, heat the avocado oil. Add the broccolini and sauté for 2 to 3 minutes. Season with the salt and pepper and transfer it to the bowl containing the spinach.

Add the cauliflower rice to the skillet and cook for 3 minutes. Add it to the serving bowl.

Top with the carrots and avocado.

Drizzle with the melted almond butter, sprinkle the cilantro on top, and serve.

Nutrition:

Calories 82 Total Fat 3.2g

Net Carbs 2.7g Protein 12.4g

Fiber 2.7g

32. Cauliflower Rice and Mushroom Risotto

Preparation Time: 20 Minutes

Cooking Time: 30 Minutes

Serving: 6

Ingredients:

Black pepper, one teaspoon

Salt, .5 teaspoon

Parsley, fresh, chopped, two tablespoons

Parmesan cheese, grated, .5 cup

Heavy cream, one cup

Cauliflower, riced, four cups

Vegetable broth, two cups divided

Mushrooms, button, one cup sliced thin

Shallot, one large, minced

Onion, one small, well diced

Garlic, minced, six cloves

Olive oil, two tablespoons

Butter, two tablespoons

Directions:

Add the olive oil and the butter together in one pan and fry the shallot, onion, and garlic for five minutes.

Pour in one cup of the vegetables broth and the mushrooms and cook for five more minutes.

To this mix and the other cup of vegetable broth and the riced cauliflower, cooking for ten minutes while stirring often.

Pour in the heavy cream, salt, pepper, parsley, and the parmesan cheese and turn the heat under the pot to low. Simmer this for ten to fifteen minutes or until the mix is thickened.

Nutrition: Calories 297 Cal

Carbs: 7.5 g Protein:7 Fat: 26 g

33. Grilled Eggplant Roll-Ups

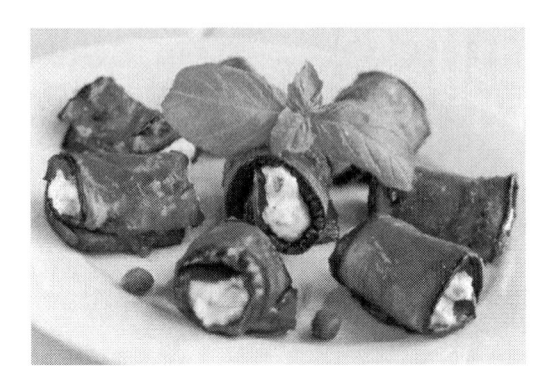

Preparation Time: 5 Minutes

Cooking Time: 8 Minutes

Servings: 8

Ingredients:

Olive oil, two tablespoons

Basil, fresh, chopped, two tablespoons

Tomato, one large

Mozzarella cheese, four ounces

Eggplant, one medium

Directions:

After cutting off both of the ends of the eggplant slice it into strips the long way about a quarter inch thick. Slice the tomato and the mozzarella very thinly and set to the side.

Brush the olive oil onto the slices of eggplant and grill them in a skillet for three minutes on each side.

When both sides are grilled lay a slice of cheese and a slice of tomato on each zucchini slice. Sprinkle all with the black pepper and the basil, then let grill for two to three minutes until the cheese begins to soften.

Remove the slices from the skillet and lie on a plate, then carefully roll each slice as far as it will roll.

Nutrition:

Calorie 59 Carbs: 4 g

Protein: 3 g Fat: 3 g

34. Eggplant Gratin with Feta Cheese

Preparation Time: 15 Minutes

Cooking Time: 40 Minutes

Servings: 6

Ingredients: Salt, .5 teaspoon

Black pepper, .5 teaspoon

Olive oil, three tablespoons

Tomato sauce, .5 cup

Gruyere cheese, .75 cup,

Basil, fresh chop, .25 cup

Chives, chopped, one tablespoon

Thyme, chopped, one teaspoon

Feta cheese, crumbled, three ounces

Heavy cream, one cup

Eggplant, two, half-inch slices

Directions:

Heat oven to 375. Lay the eggplant slices on a baking pan and coat with olive oil and sprinkle on pepper and salt and bake the slices for twenty minutes.

While they are baking put the Feta cheese and heavy cream in a pot and let boil.

Remove the cooking pot from the heat and stir in the chives and thyme and set to the side.

Spread all of the tomato sauce on the bottom of a nine by thirteen baking pan and lay the eggplant slices over the bottom.

Cover the slices with the Gruyere cheese and the basil. Add another layer with the rest of the eggplant and cover all with the heavy cream mixture. Bake for twenty minutes.

Nutrition:

Calories: 302 Cal Carbs 14 g Protein: 9 g

Fat: 24 g

35. Tofu Pesto Zoodles

Preparation Time: 5 Minutes

Cooking Time: 12 Minutes

Servings: 4

Ingredients:

2 tbsp olive oil

1 medium white onion, chopped

1 garlic clove, minced

2 (14 oz) blocks firm tofu, soaked and cubed

1 medium red bell pepper, deseeded and sliced

6 medium zucchinis, spiralized

¼ cup basil pesto, olive oil-based

Salt and freshly ground black pepper to taste

½ cup shredded Gouda cheese

2/3 cup grated Parmesan cheese

Toasted pine nuts to garnish

Directions:

Over medium fire, heat olive oil in a medium pot and sauté onion and garlic until softened and fragrant, 3 minutes.

Add tofu and cook until golden on all sides. Pour in bell pepper and cook until softened, 4 minutes.

Mix in zucchinis, pesto, salt, and black pepper. Cook for 3 minutes or until zucchinis soften slightly. Turn heat off and carefully mix in Gouda cheese to melt.

Dish into four plates, top with Parmesan cheese, pine nuts, and serve.

Nutrition:

Calories: 477 Cal Fat: 32 g

Carbs: 12.04 g Fiber: 6.6 g Protein: 20.42 g

36. Cheesy Mushroom Pie

Preparation Time: 10 Minutes

Cooking Time: 43 Minutes

Servings: 4

Ingredients:

For piecrust:

3 tbsp coconut flour

¼ cup almond flour + extra for dusting

½ tsp salt

¼ cup butter, cold and crumbled

3 tbsp swerve sugar

1 ½ tsp vanilla extract

4 whole eggs, cracked into a bowl

For filling:

2 tbsp butter

1 medium brown onion

2 garlic cloves, minced

1 green bell pepper, deseeded and diced

1 cup green beans, cut into 3 pieces each

2 cups mixed mushrooms, chopped

Salt and freshly ground black pepper to taste

¼ cup coconut cream

1/3 cup sour cream

½ cup unsweetened almond milk

2 eggs, lightly beaten

¼ tsp nutmeg powder

1 tbsp freshly chopped parsley

1 cup grated cheddar cheese

Directions:

For piecrust:

Preheat oven to 350oF and grease a pie pan with cooking spray. Set aside.

In a large bowl, combine coconut flour, almond flour, and salt.

Add butter and mix with an electric hand mixer until crumbly. Add swerve sugar, vanilla extract, and mix well. Pour in eggs one after another while mixing until formed into a ball.

Flatten dough on a chopping board, cover in plastic wrap, and refrigerate for 1 hour.

Lightly dust chopping board with almond flour, unwrap dough, and roll out into a large rectangle of ½-inch thickness. Fit dough in pie pan, and cover with parchment paper.

Pour in some baking beans and bake in oven until golden, 10 minutes. Remove after, pour out beans, remove parchment paper, and allow cooling.

For filling:

Meanwhile, melt butter in a skillet and sauté onion and garlic until softened and fragrant, 3 minutes. Add bell pepper, green beans, mushroom, salt and black pepper; cook for 5 minutes.

In a medium bowl, beat coconut cream, sour cream, almond milk, and eggs. Season with salt, black pepper, and nutmeg. Stir in parsley and cheddar cheese.

Spread mushroom mixture in baked crust and top with cheese filling.

Bake until golden on top and cheese melted, 20 to 25 minutes.

Remove; allow cooling for 10 minutes, slice, and serve.

Nutrition:

Calories: 527 Cal

Fat: 43.58 g

Carbs: 8.73 g

Fiber: 2.2 g

Protein: 21.3 g

37. Meatless Florentine Pizza

Preparation Time: 10 Minutes

Cooking Time: 25 Minutes

Servings: 2

Ingredients:

For pizza crust:

6 eggs

1 tsp Italian seasoning

1 cup shredded provolone cheese

For topping:

2/3 cup tomato sauce

2 cups baby spinach, wilted

½ cup grated mozzarella cheese

1 (7 oz) can sliced mushrooms, drained

4 eggs

Olive oil for drizzling

Directions:

For pizza crust:

Preheat oven to 400o F and line a pizza pan with parchment paper. Set aside.

Crack eggs into a medium bowl and whisk in Italian seasoning and provolone cheese.

Spread mixture on pizza pan and bake until golden, 10 minutes. Remove and allow cooling for 2 minutes.

For pizza:

Increase oven's temperature to 450o F.

Spread tomato sauce on crust, top with spinach, mozzarella cheese, and mushrooms. Bake for 8 minutes.

Crack eggs on top and continue baking until eggs set, 2 minutes.

Remove, slice, and serve.

Nutrition:

Calories: 646 Cal Fat: 39.19 g

Carbs: 8.42 g Fiber: 3.5 g Protein: 36.87 g

38. Margherita Pizza with Cauliflower Crust

Preparation Time: 8 Minutes

Cooking Time: 30 Minutes

Servings: 2

Ingredients:

For pizza crust:

2 cups cauliflower rice

4 eggs

¼ cup shredded Monterey Jack cheese

¼ cup shredded Parmesan cheese

½ tsp Italian seasoning

Salt and freshly ground black pepper to taste

For topping:

6 tbsp unsweetened tomato sauce

1 small red onion, thinly sliced

2 ½ oz cremini mushrooms, sliced

1 tsp dried oregano

½ cup cottage cheese

½ tbsp. olive oil

A handful fresh basil

Directions:

For pizza crust:

Preheat oven to 400o F and line a baking sheet with parchment paper.

Pour cauliflower into a safe microwave bowl, sprinkle with 1 tablespoon of water, cover with plastic wrap and microwave for 1 to 2 minutes or until softened. Remove and allow cooling.

Pour cauliflower into a cheesecloth and squeeze out as much liquid. Transfer to a mixing bowl.

Crack in eggs, add cheeses, Italian seasoning, salt, and black pepper. Mix until well-combined.

Spread mixture on baking sheet and bake in oven until golden, 15 minutes.

Remove from oven and allow cooling for 2 minutes.

For topping:

Spread tomato sauce on pizza crust, scatter onion and mushrooms on top, sprinkle with oregano, and add cottage cheese. Drizzle with olive oil and bake until golden, 15 minutes.

Remove, top with basil, slice and serve.

Nutrition:

Calories: 290 Cal Fat: 22.58 g

Carbs: 6.62 g Fiber: 5.8 g

Protein: 12.81 g

39. Almond Tofu Loaf

Preparation Time: 10 Minutes

Cooking Time: 1 Hour

Servings: 4

Ingredients:

3 tbsp olive oil + extra for brushing

4 garlic cloves, minced

2 white onions, finely chopped

1 lb. firm tofu, pressed and cubed

2 tbsp coconut aminos

¾ cup chopped almonds

Salt and freshly ground black pepper

1 tbsp dried mixed herbs

½ tsp erythritol

¼ cup golden flax seed meal

1 tbsp sesame seeds

1 cup chopped mixed bell peppers

½ cup tomato sauce

Directions:

Preheat oven to 350oF and lightly brush an 8 x 4-inch loaf pan with olive oil. Set aside.

In a medium bowl, combine olive oil, garlic, onion, tofu, coconut aminos, almonds, salt, black pepper, mixed herbs, erythritol, golden flax seed meal, sesame seeds, and bell peppers, and mix well.

Fit mixture in loaf pan, spread tomato sauce on top, and bake in oven for 45 minutes to 1 hour.

Remove pan and turn tofu loaf over onto a chopping board.

Slice and serve with garden green salad.

Nutrition:

Calories: 432 Cal

Fat: 31.38 g

Carbs: 8.74 g

Fiber: 6.2 g

Protein: 24.36 g

40. Kale and Mushroom Biryani

Preparation Time: 15 Minutes

Cooking Time: 46 Minutes

Servings: 4

Ingredients:

6 cups cauli rice

2 tbsp water

Salt and freshly ground black pepper

3 tbsp ghee

3 medium white onions, chopped

1 tsp ginger puree

1 tbsp turmeric powder + more for dusting

2 cups chopped tomatoes

1 red chili, finely chopped

1 tbsp tomato puree

1 cup sliced cremini mushrooms

1 cup diced paneer cheese

1 cup kale, chopped

1/3 cup water

1 cup plain yogurt

¼ cup chopped cilantro

Olive oil for drizzling

Directions:

Preheat oven to 400o F.

Pour cauliflower rice into a safe microwave bowl, drizzle with water, cover with plastic wrap, and microwave for 1 minute or until softened. Remove and season with salt and black pepper. Set aside.

Melt ghee in a casserole pan and sauté onion, ginger, and turmeric powder. Cook until fragrant, 5 minutes.

Add tomatoes, red chili, and tomato puree; cook until tomatoes soften, 5 minutes.

Stir in mushrooms, paneer cheese, kale, and water; season with salt and black pepper and simmer until mushrooms soften, 10 minutes. Turn heat off and stir in yogurt.

Spoon half of stew into a bowl and set aside. Sprinkle half of cilantro on remaining stew in casserole pan, top with half of cauli rice, and dust with turmeric. Repeat layering a second time with remaining ingredients.

Drizzle with olive oil and bake until golden and crisp on top, 25 minutes.

Remove; allow cooling, and serve with coconut chutney.

Nutrition:

Calories: 346 Cal Fat: 21.48 g

Carbs: 8.63 g Fiber: 6.6 g

Protein: 16.01 g

41. Mushroom Pizza Bowls with Avocado & Cilantro

Preparation Time: 15 Minutes

Cooking Time: 17 Minutes

Servings: 4

Ingredients: 1 ½ cups broccoli rice

2 tbsp water

Olive oil for brushing

2 cups unsweetened pizza sauce

1 cup grated Gruyere cheese

1 cup grated mozzarella cheese

2 large tomatoes, chopped

½ cup sliced cremini mushrooms

1 small red onion, chopped

1 tsp dried basil

Salt and freshly ground black pepper to taste

1 avocado, halved, pitted, and chopped

¼ cup chopped parsley

Directions:

Preheat oven to 400o F.

Pour broccoli rice into a safe microwave bowl, drizzle with water, and steam in microwave for 1 to 2 minutes. Remove, fluff with a fork, and set aside.

Lightly brush the inner parts of four medium ramekins with olive oil and spread in half of pizza sauce. Top with half of broccoli rice and half of cheeses.

In a bowl, combine tomatoes, mushrooms, onion, basil, salt, and black pepper. Spoon half of mixture into ramekins and top with half of cheeses. Repeat layering a second time making sure to finish off with cheeses.

Bake until cheese melts and golden on top, 15 minutes.

Remove ramekins and top with avocados and parsley.

Allow cooling for 3 minutes and serve.

Nutrition:

Calories: 378 Cal Fat: 22.54 g

Carbs: 12.27 g Fiber: 8.9 g Protein: 20.68 g

42. Pistachios and Cheese Stuffed Zucchinis

Preparation Time: 15 Minutes

Cooking Time: 17 Minutes

Servings: 4

Ingredients: 1 cup rice broccoli

¼ cup vegetable broth

4 medium zucchinis, halved

2 tbsp olive oil + more for drizzling

1 ¼ cup diced tomatoes

1 medium red onion, chopped

¼ cup pine nuts ¼ cup chopped pistachios

4 tbsp chopped parsley

1 tbsp smoked paprika

1 tbsp balsamic vinegar

Salt and freshly ground black pepper to taste

1 cup grated Parmesan cheese

Directions:

Preheat oven to 350oF.

Pour broccoli rice and vegetable broth in a medium pot and cook over medium heat until softened, 2 minutes. Turn heat off, fluff broccoli rice, and allow cooling.

Scoop flesh out of zucchini halves, chop pulp and set aside. Brush zucchini boats with some olive oil. Set aside.

In a medium bowl, combine broccoli rice, tomatoes, red onion, pine nuts, pistachios, parsley, paprika, balsamic vinegar, zucchini pulp, salt, and black pepper.

Spoon mixture into zucchini boats, drizzle with more olive oil, and cover top with Parmesan cheese.

Place filled zucchinis on a baking sheet and bake until cheese melts and is golden, 15 minutes.

Remove, allow cooling, and serve.

Nutrition: Calories: 330 CalFat: 28.12 g

Carbs: 10.62 g Fiber: 5.4 g Protein: 12.3 g

43. Soy Chorizo-Asparagus Bowl

Preparation Time: 15 Minutes

Cooking Time: 15 Minutes

Servings: 4

Ingredients:

1 lb. soy chorizo, cubed

1 lb. asparagus, trimmed and halved

1 cup green beans, trimmed

1 cup chopped mixed bell peppers

2 red onions, cut into wedges

1 head medium broccoli, cut into florets

2 rosemary sprigs

Salt and freshly ground black pepper to taste

4 tbsp olive oil

1 tbsp maple (sugar-free) syrup

1 lemon, juiced

Directions:

Preheat oven to 400o F.

On a baking tray, spread soy chorizo, asparagus, green beans, bell peppers, onions, broccoli, and rosemary. Season with salt, black pepper, and drizzle with olive oil and maple syrup. Rub spices into vegetables.

Bake until vegetables soften and light brown around the edges, 15 minutes.

Dish vegetables into serving bowls, drizzle with lemon juice, and serve warm.

Nutrition:

Calories: 300 Cal Fat: 18.55 g Carbs: 12.5 g

Fiber: 9.2 g Protein: 14.87 g

44. Creamy Brussels Sprouts Bowls

Preparation Time: 10 Minutes

Cooking Time: 30 Minutes

Servings: 4

Ingredients: 1 tablespoon olive oil

1-pound Brussels sprouts, trimmed and halved

1 cup coconut cream

½ teaspoon chili powder

½ teaspoon garam masala

½ teaspoon garlic powder

A pinch of salt and black pepper

1 tablespoon lime juice

Directions: 2In a roasting pan, combine the sprouts with the cream, chili powder and the other ingredients, toss, introduce in the oven at 380 degrees F and bake for 30 minutes. Divide into bowls and serve for lunch.

Nutrition: Calories: 219 Cal Fat: 18.3 g

Fiber: 5.7 g Carbs: 14.1 Protein: 5.4 g

45. Green Beans and Radishes Bake

Preparation Time: 10 Minutes

Cooking Time: 25 Minutes

Servings: 4

Ingredients:

2 tablespoons olive oil

1-pound green beans, trimmed and halved

2 cups radishes, sliced

1 cup coconut cream

1 teaspoon sweet paprika

1 cup cashew cheese, shredded

Salt and black pepper to the taste

1 tablespoon chives, chopped

Directions:

In a roasting pan, combine the green beans with the radishes and the other ingredients except the cheese and toss.

Sprinkle the cheese on top, introduce in the oven at 375 degrees F and bake for 25 minutes.

Divide the mix between plates and serve.

Nutrition: Calories: 130 Cal

Fat: 1 g Fiber: 0.4 g

Carbs: 1 g Protein: 0.1 g

46. Avocado and Radish Bowls

Preparation Time: 10 Minutes

Cooking Time: 0

Servings: 4

Ingredients:

2 cups radishes, halved

2 avocados, peeled, pitted and roughly cubed

2 tablespoons coconut cream

2 tablespoons balsamic vinegar

1 tablespoon green onion, chopped

1 teaspoon chili powder

1 cup baby spinach

Salt and black pepper to the taste

Directions:

In a bowl, combine the radishes with the avocados and the other ingredients, toss, divide into smaller bowls and serve for lunch.

Nutrition:

Calories: 340 Cal

Fat: 23

Fiber: 3 g

Carbs: 6 g

Protein: 5 g

47. Celery and Radish Soup

Preparation Time: 10 Minutes

Cooking Time: 20 Minutes

Servings: 4

Ingredients:

½ pound radishes, cut into quarters

2 celery stalks, chopped

2 tablespoons olive oil

4 scallions, chopped

1 teaspoon fennel seeds, crushed

1 teaspoon coriander, dried

6 cups vegetable stock

Salt and black pepper to the taste

6 garlic cloves, minced

1 tablespoon chives, chopped

Directions:

Heat up a pot with the oil over medium heat, add the celery, scallions and the garlic and sauté for 5 minutes.

Add the radishes and the other ingredients, bring to a boil, cover and simmer for 15 minutes.

Divide into soup bowls and serve.

Nutrition:

Calories: 120 Cal Fat: 2 g

Fiber: 1 g Carbs: 3 g Protein: 10 g

48. Lime Avocado and Cucumber Soup

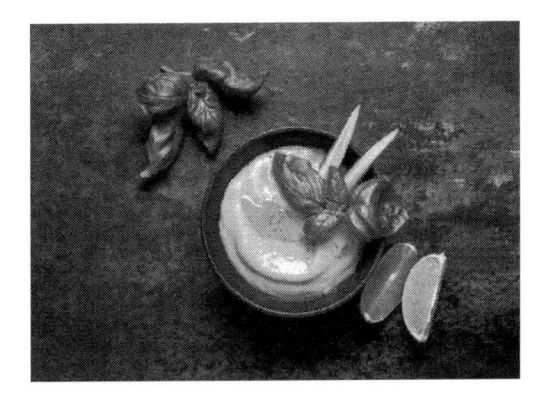

Preparation Time: 5 Minutes

Cooking Time: 0 Minutes

Servings: 4

Ingredients: 1 tablespoon olive oil

2 avocados, pitted, peeled and roughly cubed

2 cucumbers, sliced   4 cups vegetable stock

Salt and black pepper to the taste

¼ teaspoon lemon zest, grated

1 tablespoon white vinegar

1 cup scallions, chopped

¼ cup cilantro, chopped

Directions: In a blender, combine the avocados with the cucumbers and the other ingredients, pulse well, divide into bowls and serve for lunch.

Nutrition: Calories: 100 Cal

Fat: 10 g Fiber: 2 g Carbs: 5 g Protein: 8 g

49. Avocado and Kale Soup

Preparation Time: 5 Minutes

Cooking Time: 7 Minutes

Servings: 4

Ingredients:

4 cups kale, torn

1 teaspoon turmeric powder

1 avocado, pitted, peeled and sliced

4 cups vegetable stock

Juice of 1 lime

2 garlic cloves, minced

1 tablespoon chives, chopped

Salt and black pepper to the taste

Directions:

In a pot, combine the kale with the avocado and the other ingredients, bring to a simmer, cook over medium heat for 7 minutes, blend using an immersion blender, divide into bowls and serve.

Nutrition:

Calories: 234 Cal

Fat: 4 g

Carbs: 7 g

Protein :12

50. Spinach and Cucumber Salad

Preparation Time: 5 Minutes

Cooking Time: 0

Servings: 4

Ingredients:

1-pound cucumber, sliced

2 cups baby spinach

1 tablespoon chili powder

2 tablespoons olive oil

¼ cup cilantro, chopped

2 tablespoons lemon juice

Salt and black pepper to the taste

Directions:

In a large salad bowl, combine the cucumber with the spinach and the other ingredients, toss and serve for lunch.

Nutrition:

Calories: 140 Cal

Fat: 4 g

Fiber: 2 g

Carbs: 4 g

Protein: 5 g

Snack Recipes

51. Nori Snack Rolls

Preparation Time: 5 Minutes

Cooking Time: 10 Minutes

Servings: 4

Ingredients

2 tablespoons almond, cashew, peanut, or other nut butter

2 tablespoons tamari, or soy sauce

4 standard nori sheets

1 mushroom, sliced

1 tablespoon pickled ginger

½ cup grated carrots

Directions

Preheat the oven to 350°F.

Mix together the nut butter and tamari until smooth and very thick. Lay out a nori sheet, rough side up, the long way.

Spread a thin line of the tamari mixture on the far end of the nori sheet, from side to side. Lay the mushroom slices, ginger, and carrots in a line at the other end (the end closest to you).

Fold the vegetables inside the nori, rolling toward the tahini mixture, which will seal the roll. Repeat to make 4 rolls.

Put on a baking sheet and bake for 8 to 10 minutes, or until the rolls are slightly browned and crispy at the ends. Let the rolls cool for a few minutes, then slice each roll into 3 smaller pieces.

Nutrition

Calories: 79 Cal Fat: 5 g

Carbs: 6 gFiber: 2 g Protein: 4 g

52. Risotto Bites

Preparation Time: 15 Minutes

Cooking Time: 20 Minutes

Servings: 12

Ingredients

½ cup panko bread crumbs

1 teaspoon paprika

1 teaspoon chipotle powder or ground cayenne pepper

1½ cups cold Green Pea Risotto

Nonstick cooking spray

Directions

Preheat the oven to 425°F.

Line a baking sheet with parchment paper.

On a large plate, combine the panko, paprika, and chipotle powder. Set aside.

Roll 2 tablespoons of the risotto into a ball.

Gently roll in the bread crumbs, and place on the prepared baking sheet. Repeat to make a total of 12 balls.

Spritz the tops of the risotto bites with nonstick cooking spray and bake for 15 to 20 minutes, until they begin to brown. Cool completely before storing in a large airtight container in a single layer (add a piece of parchment paper for a second layeror in a plastic freezer bag.

Nutrition:

Calories: 100 Cal

Fat: 2 g

Protein: 6 g

Carbs: 17 g

Fiber: 5 g

53. Jicama and Guacamole

Preparation Time: 15 Minutes

Cooking Time: 0

Servings: 4

Ingredients

juice of 1 lime, or 1 tablespoon prepared lime juice

2 hass avocados, peeled, pits removed, and cut into cubes

½ teaspoon sea salt

½ red onion, minced

1 garlic clove, minced

¼ cup chopped cilantro (optional

1 jicama bulb, peeled and cut into matchsticks

Directions

In a medium bowl, squeeze the lime juice over the top of the avocado and sprinkle with salt.

Lightly mash the avocado with a fork. Stir in the onion, garlic, and cilantro, if using.

Serve with slices of jicama to dip in guacamole.

To store, place plastic wrap over the bowl of guacamole and refrigerate. The guacamole will keep for about 2 days.

Nutrition:

Calories: 130 Cal Fat: 2 g Protein: 5 g

Carbs: 13 g Fiber: 5 g

54. Curried Tofu "Egg Salad" Pitas

Preparation Time: 15 Minutes

Cooking Time: 0 Minutes

Servings: 4 Sandwiches

Ingredients

1-pound extra-firm tofu, drained and patted dry

1/2 cup vegan mayonnaise, homemade or store-bought

1/4 cup chopped mango chutney, homemade or store-bought

2 teaspoons Dijon mustard

1 tablespoon hot or mild curry powder

1 teaspoon salt

1/8 teaspoon ground cayenne

¾ cup shredded carrots

2 celery ribs, minced

1/4 cup minced red onion

8 small Boston or other soft lettuce leaves

4 (7-inch whole wheat pita breads, halved

Directions

Crumble the tofu and place it in a large bowl. Add the mayonnaise, chutney, mustard, curry powder, salt, and cayenne, and stir well until thoroughly mixed.

Add the carrots, celery, and onion and stir to combine. Refrigerate for 30 minutes to allow the flavors to blend.

Tuck a lettuce leaf inside each pita pocket, spoon some tofu mixture on top of the lettuce, and serve.

Nutrition:

Calories: 200 CalFat: 3 g Protein: 9 g

Carbs: 11 g Fiber: 8 g

55. Garden Patch Sandwiches on Multigrain Bread

Preparation Time: 15 Minutes

Cooking Time: 0 Minutes

Servings: 4 Sandwiches

Ingredients

1 pound extra-firm tofu, drained and patted dry

1 medium red bell pepper, finely chopped

1 celery rib, finely chopped

3 green onions, minced

1/4 cup shelled sunflower seeds

1/2 cup vegan mayonnaise, homemade or store-bought

1/2 teaspoon salt

1/2 teaspoon celery salt

1/4 teaspoon freshly ground black pepper

8 slices whole grain bread

4 (1/4-inchslices ripe tomato

4 lettuce leaves

Directions

Crumble the tofu and place it in a large bowl. Add the bell pepper, celery, green onions, and sunflower seeds. Stir in the mayonnaise, salt, celery salt, and pepper and mix until well combined.

Toast the bread, if desired. Spread the mixture evenly onto 4 slices of the bread. Top each with a tomato slice, lettuce leaf, and the remaining bread. Cut the sandwiches diagonally in half and serve.

Nutrition:

Calories: 234 Cal Fat: 6 g

Protein: 3 g Carbs: 12 g Fiber: 9 g

56. Garden Salad Wraps

Preparation Time: 15 Minutes

Cooking Time: 10 Minutes

Servings: 4 Wraps

Ingredients 6 tablespoons olive oil

1-pound extra-firm tofu, drained, patted dry, and cut into 1/2-inch strips

1 tablespoon soy sauce

1/4 cup apple cider vinegar

1 teaspoon yellow or spicy brown mustard

1/2 teaspoon salt

1/4 teaspoon freshly ground black pepper

3 cups shredded romaine lettuce

3 ripe Roma tomatoes, finely chopped

1 large carrot, shredded

1 medium English cucumber, peeled and chopped

1/3 cup minced red onion

1/4 cup sliced pitted green olives

4 (10-inchwhole-grain flour tortillas or lavash flatbread

Directions

In a large skillet, heat 2 tablespoons of the oil over medium heat. Add the tofu and cook until golden brown, about 10 minutes. Sprinkle with soy sauce and set aside to cool. In a small bowl, combine the vinegar, mustard, salt, and pepper with the remaining 4 tablespoons oil, stirring to blend well. Set aside. In a large bowl, combine the lettuce, tomatoes, carrot, cucumber, onion, and olives. Pour on the dressing and toss to coat. To assemble wraps, place 1 tortilla on a work surface and spread with about one-quarter of the salad. Place a few strips of tofu on the tortilla and roll up tightly. Slice in half

Nutrition: Calories: 200 Cal Fat: 5 g

Protein: 6 g Carbs: 7 g Fiber: 7 g

57. Black Sesame Wonton Chips

Preparation Time: 5 Minutes

Cooking Time: 5 Minutes

Servings: 6

Ingredients

12 Vegan Wonton Wrappers

Toasted sesame oil

1/3 cup black sesame seeds

Salt

Directions

Preheat the oven to 450°F. Lightly oil a baking sheet and set aside. Cut the wonton wrappers in half crosswise, brush them with sesame oil, and arrange them in a single layer on the prepared baking sheet.

Sprinkle wonton wrappers with the sesame seeds and salt to taste, and bake until crisp and golden brown, 5 to 7 minutes. Cool completely before serving. These are best eaten on the day they are made but, once cooled, they can be covered and stored at room temperature for 1 to 2 days.

Nutrition:

Calories: 150 Cal

Fat: 2 g

Protein : 8 g

Carbs: 11 g

Fiber: 9 g

58. Marinated Mushroom Wraps

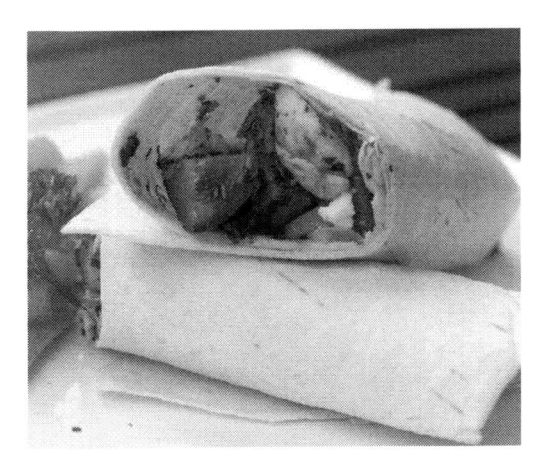

Preparation time: 15 minutes

cooking time: 0 minutes

servings: 2

Ingredients

3 tablespoons soy sauce

3 tablespoons fresh lemon juice

1 1/2 tablespoons toasted sesame oil

2 portobello mushroom caps, cut into 1/4-inch strips

1 ripe Hass avocado, pitted and peeled

2 (10-inchwhole-grain flour tortillas

2 cups fresh baby spinach leaves

1 medium red bell pepper, cut into 1/4-inch strips

1 ripe tomato, chopped

Salt and freshly ground black pepper

Directions

In a medium bowl, combine the soy sauce, 2 tablespoons of the lemon juice, and the oil. Add the portobello strips, toss to combine, and marinate for 1 hour or overnight. Drain the mushrooms and set aside.

Mash the avocado with the remaining 1 tablespoon of lemon juice.

To assemble wraps, place 1 tortilla on a work surface and spread with some of the mashed avocado. Top with a layer of baby spinach leaves. In the lower third of each tortilla, arrange strips of the soaked mushrooms and some of the bell pepper strips. Sprinkle with the tomato and salt and black pepper to taste. Roll up tightly and cut in half diagonally. Repeat with the remaining Ingredients and serve.

Nutrition:

Calories: 143 Cal

Fat: 3g

Protein: 16 g

Carbs: 7 g

Fiber: 3 g

59. Tamari Toasted Almonds

Preparation Time: 2 Minutes

Cooking Time: 8 Minutes

Servings: 1

Ingredients

½ cup raw almonds, or sunflower seeds

2 tablespoons tamari, or soy sauce

1 teaspoon toasted sesame oil

Directions

Heat a dry skillet to medium-high heat, then add the almonds, stirring very frequently to keep them from burning. Once the almonds are toasted, 7 to 8 minutes for almonds, or 3 to 4 minutes for sunflower seeds, pour the tamari and sesame oil into the hot skillet and stir to coat.

You can turn off the heat, and as the almonds cool the tamari mixture will stick to and dry on the nuts.

Nutrition:

Calories: 89 Cal

fat: 8 g

Carbs: 3 g

Fiber: 2 g

Protein: 4 g

60. Avocado and Tempeh Bacon Wraps

Preparation Time: 10 Minutes

Cooking Time: 8 Minutes

Servings: 4

Ingredients   2 tablespoons olive oil

8 ounces tempeh bacon, homemade or store-bought

4 (10-inchsoft flour tortillas or lavash flat bread

1/4 cup vegan mayonnaise, homemade or store-bought - 4 large lettuce leaves

2 ripe Hass avocados, pitted, peeled, and cut into 1/4-inch slices

1 large ripe tomato, cut into 1/4-inch slices

Directions

In a large skillet, heat the oil over medium heat. Add the tempeh bacon and cook until browned on both sides, about 8 minutes. Remove from the heat and set aside.

Place 1 tortilla on a work surface. Spread with some of t he mayonnaise and one-fourth of the lettuce and tomatoes.

Pit, peel, and thinly slice the avocado and place the slices on top of the tomato. Add the reserved tempeh bacon and roll up tightly. Repeat with remaining Ingredients and serve.

Nutrition: Calories: 132 Cal Fat: 1 g

Protein: 8 g Carbs: 12 g Fiber: 2 g

61. Kale Chips

Preparation Time: 5 Minutes

Cooking Time: 25 Minutes

Servings: 2

Ingredients

1 large bunch kale

1 tablespoon extra-virgin olive oil

1/2 teaspoon chipotle powder

1/2 teaspoon smoked paprika

1/4 teaspoon salt

Directions

Preheat the oven to 275°F.

Line a large baking sheet with parchment paper. In a large bowl, stem the kale and tear it into bite-size pieces. Add the olive oil, chipotle powder, smoked paprika, and salt.

Toss the kale with tongs or your hands, coating each piece well.

Spread the kale over the parchment paper in a single layer.

Bake for 25 minutes, turning halfway through, until crisp.

Cool for 10 to 15 minutes before dividing and storing in 2 airtight containers.

Nutrition:

Calories: 144 Cal Fat: 7 g Protein: 5 g

Carbs: 18 g Fiber: 3 g

62. Tempeh-Pimiento Cheese Ball

Preparation Time: 5 Minutes

Cooking Time: 30 Minutes

Servings: 8

Ingredients ¾ cup chopped pecans

8 ounces tempeh, cut into 1/2-inch pieces

1 (2-ounce jar chopped pimientos, drained

1/4 cup nutritional yeast

1/4 cup vegan mayonnaise, homemade or store-bought

2 tablespoons soy sauce

Directions

In a medium saucepan of simmering water, cook the tempeh for 30 minutes. Set aside to cool. In a food processor, combine the cooled tempeh, pimientos, nutritional yeast, mayo, and soy sauce. Process until smooth. Transfer the tempeh mixture to a bowl and refrigerate until firm and chilled, at least 2 hours or overnight. In a dry skillet, toast the pecans over medium heat until lightly toasted, about 5 minutes. Set aside to cool. Shape the temp eh mixture into a ball, and roll it in the pecans, pressin g the nuts slightly into the tempeh mixture so they stick. Refrigerate for at least 1 hour before serving. If not using right away, cover and keep refrigerated until needed. Properly stored, it will keep for 2 to 3 days.

Nutrition: Calories: 188 Cal Fat: 3 g

Protein: 4 g Carbs: 19 g Fiber: 8 g

63. Seaweed Crackers

Preparation Time: 10 Minutes

Cooking Time: 24 Hours

Servings: 4

Ingredients:

1/2 cup flax seeds

1/2 cup golden flax seeds

1 1/2 cups water

2 tablespoon gluten-free tamari

2 nori sheets, broken up

Directions:

Soak tamari and flaxseeds in water in a bowl for 1 hour.

Add nori to this water and mix well.

Add 1 tablespoon of this mixture per cracker over Teflon sheet.

Place this sheet in the dehydrator and cook for 24 hours at 110 degrees F.

Flip the crackers after 12 hours.

Serve fresh.

Nutrition:

Calories: 221 Cal

Fat: 7.3 g Carbs: 3 g

Protein: 14.2 g

64. Sesame Tamari Almonds

Preparation Time: 10 Minutes

Cooking Time: 5 Minutes

Servings: 4

Ingredients:

4 teaspoons toasted sesame oil

3 tablespoons low sodium gluten-free tamari

2 pinches of salt

1/4 teaspoon swerve

2 cups of raw almonds

2 tablespoons sesame seeds

Directions:

Mix tamari, salt, sesame oil and stevia in a small bowl.

Toast almonds in a nonstick skillet then add sesame tamari mixture.

Stir cook for 5 minutes.

Drizzle sesame seeds over them.

Enjoy fresh.

Nutrition:

Calories: 152 Cal

Fat: 31.3 g

Carbs: 2.7 g

Protein: 3.7 g

65. Edamame Avocado Hummus

Preparation Time: 10 Minutes

Cooking Time: 0

Servings: 6

Ingredients:

1 clove garlic minced

12 oz. bag shelled edamame soybeans

1/4 cup tahini

1/4 cup lemon juice

1/2 cup avocado

1/4 cup water or more if desired

2 tablespoons olive oil

salt and pepper

Directions:

Add everything to a blender jug.

Pulse well until smooth.

Serve the hummus with low car crackers.

Nutrition:

Calories: 166 Cal

Fat: 11.4 g

Carbohydrates: 6.6 g

Protein: 2.4 g

66. Pizza Cheese Ball

Preparation Time: 10 Minutes

Cooking Time: 0

Servings: 4

Ingredients: 1 (8 ounces) cream cheese

1 (10 ounces) vegetarian mozzarella

1/4 cup sun-dried tomatoes

1/4 cup green olives

1 teaspoon basil 1 teaspoon oregano

1/2 teaspoon garlic powder

1/2 teaspoon onion powder

1 teaspoon red pepper flakes

Salt and pepper 1/4 cup walnuts chopped

Directions:

Slice the mozzarella block into thin strips. Grind walnuts in a food processor and spread them in a plate.

Blend all the remaining ingredients for the ball in the blender.

Make small balls out of this mixture then roll them in walnuts.

Wrap the cheese strips over the cheese balls.

Enjoy fresh.

Nutrition:

Calories: 94 Cal Fat: 7 g

Carbs: 5 g Protein: 1 g

67. Tahini Keto Bagels

Preparation Time: 10 minutes

Cooking Time: 40 minutes

Servings: 4

Ingredients: 1/2 cup ground flax seed

1/2 cup tahini 1/4 cup psyllium husks

1 cup of water 1 teaspoon baking powder

pinch of salt

sesame seeds for garnish

Directions:

Let your oven preheat at 375 degrees F.

Whisk psyllium husk with baking powder, flaxseeds, and salt in a mixing bowl.

Mix tahini with water in a separate bowl until well combined.

Add the husk mixture to make a dough. Knead well over the working surface.

Make 4 inches in diameter patties with ¼ inch thickness.

Place the prepared patties on the baking tray and drizzle sesame seeds over them.

Bake the patties for 40 minutes in the set oven until golden brown.

Enjoy fresh.

Nutrition: Calories: 79 Cal Fat: 4.3 g

Carbs: 7.1 g Protein: 2.6 g

68. Zucchini Nests

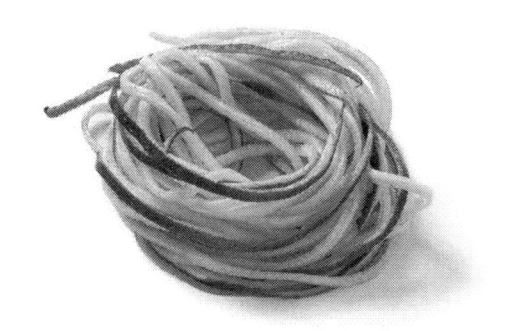

Preparation Time: 10 Minutes

Cooking Time: 10 Minutes

Servings: 4

Ingredients:

3 large zucchinis, spiralized

1 teaspoon of sea salt

1/4 teaspoon garlic powder

1/4 teaspoon onion powder

1/8 teaspoon ground black pepper

4 large eggs

Coconut oil, for greasing

Directions:

Pass the zucchini through the spiralizer cutter to make its thin noodles.

Place the noodles in a colander and sprinkle salt over th em then leave them for 20 minutes.

Let your oven preheat at 400 degrees and grease a muffin tin with coconut oil.

Squeeze all the water out the noodles by pressing them firmly.

Mix black pepper, onion powder and garlic powder in a large bowl.

Toss in zucchini noodles and mix well to coat.

Divide the noodles into the muffin cups and make a nest at the center of each muffin cup.

Crack one egg at the center of each nest.

Drizzle salt and pepper on top.

Bake for 10 minutes until it's done.

Serve fresh.

Nutrition: Calories: 155 Cal

Fat: 2.1 g Carbs: 5.9 g Protein: 12.6 g

69. Low Carb Bibimbap

Preparation Time: 10 Minutes

Cooking Time: 10 Minutes

Servings: 4

Ingredients: 1 tablespoon soy sauce

2 tablespoons rice vinegar

7 oz tempeh, sliced into squares

1 small red bell pepper, in strips

4-6 broccoli florets, in thin spears

1 carrot, grated 1/2 cucumber, in strips

10 oz raw cauliflower, riced

2 tablespoons chili paste

2 tablespoons rice vinegar

1 tablespoon soy sauce

1 teaspoon sesame oil

concentrated liquid sweetener to taste

2 tablespoons sesame seeds

Directions:

Whisk soy sauce with vinegar in a bowl then toss in tempeh squares.

Let them sit for 1 minute and meanwhile dice the vegetables. Warm oil in a skillet and sauté tempeh in it for 4 minutes on medium heat.

Transfer the tempeh to a plate then add broccoli, carrots, and peppers. Cover the skillet and cook for 2 minutes. Sauté cauliflower rice in a separate pan until soft.

Mix soy sauce with chili paste, oil, and sweetener in a small bowl.

Toss cauliflower rice with tempeh, peppers, broccoli, carrot, and cucumber in a salad bowl.

Stir in chili paste mixture and mix well to coat. Garnish with sesame seeds.

Enjoy fresh.

Nutrition: Calories: 164 Cal

Fat: 10.3 g Carbohydrates: 4 g Protein: 1.4 g

70. Walnut Carrot Bombs

Preparation Time: 10 Minutes

Cooking Time: 45 Minutes

Servings: 6

Ingredients: 1/2 cup raw walnut

3 medium carrots, peeled and grated

2 cloves garlic, minced

Salt and pepper, to taste

1 tablespoon cream cheese

1 tablespoon heavy cream

1/2 cup shredded Parmesan cheese

Directions:

Let your oven preheat at 350 degrees F and layer a muffin tin with cooking oil. Grate carrots by grinding them in a food processor on high speed. Add walnuts and grind again to make a crumbly mixture.

Stir in cheese, cream cheese, cream, salt, garlic, and black pepper. Blend again until evenly mixed. Make small golf ball sized balls out of this mixture.

Place each ball in the muffin cups and bake them for 45 minutes until golden brown.

Allow it to cool for 5 minutes approximately then serve fresh.

Nutrition: Calories: 118 Cal

Fat: 18.3 g Carbs: 9 g Protein: 5.1 g

71. Nutty Zucchini Salad

Preparation Time: 10 Minutes

Cooking Time: 3 Minutes

Servings: 2

Ingredients:

1/4 cup pine nuts

2 tablespoons butter

1 large zucchini, julienned

Salt to taste

2 tablespoons Parmesan cheese, grated

Directions:

Add and melt butter in a large skillet over medium heat then toss in pine nuts.

Stir cook for 3 minutes until golden brown.

Add zucchini and sauté for few seconds then add salt to adjust seasoning.

Garnish with parmesan then serve fresh.

Nutrition:

Calories: 102 Cal

Fat: 17.3 g

Carbs: 6.1 g

Protein: 1.2 g

72. Kale Pate Spread

Preparation Time: 10 Minutes

Cooking Time: 7 Minutes

Servings: 6

Ingredients:

6 cups green kale, chopped

1 tablespoon olive oil

½ cup raw organic sesame seeds

½ cup extra-virgin olive oil

8 green onions, green parts only

3 tablespoon apple cider vinegar

1 ¼ teaspoon grey sea salt

Directions:

Mix kale with a tablespoon of olive oil and cook it under the lid for 7 minutes in a skillet on low heat.

Transfer the kale to a food processor along with all the remaining ingredients.

Pulse to make a smooth mixture then transfer it to a mason jar.

Refrigerate and store for 4 days.

Serve it with low carb crackers.

Nutrition:

Calories: 61 Cal Fat: 21.2 g

Carbs: 6 g Protein: 4.1 g

73. Smoked Almonds

Preparation Time: 5 Minutes

Cooking Time: 45 Minutes

Servings: 10

Ingredients: 1-pound raw almonds

2 tablespoons grass-fed butter, melted

2 tablespoons liquid smoke

2 tablespoons Worcestershire sauce

1 tablespoon salt

Directions:

Preheat the oven to 200°F. Line a baking dish with aluminum foil.

Put the almonds in a large mixing bowl and set aside.

In a sm all bowl, mix together the butter, liquid smoke, and Worcestershire sauce.

Pour the mixture over the almonds and stir. Sprinkle in the salt and mix again.

Spread the almonds evenly on the prepared baking dish and place in the oven.

Coo k for 45 minutes, stirring well every 10 minutes. Once cooked, transfer the nuts to paper towels to drain. When cool, store in an airtight container until ready to serve.

Nutrition:

Calories: 305 Cal Fat: 25 g

Protein: 10 g Carbs: 10 g Fiber: 6 g

74. Roasted Garlic Mushrooms

Preparation Time: 5 Minutes

Cooking Time: 25 Minutes

Servings: 4

Ingredients: ½ teaspoon salt

Nonstick cooking spray

1⅓ pounds cremini mushrooms

6 garlic cloves, minced

3 tablespoons avocado oil

3 tablespoons Parmesan cheese

¼ teaspoon freshly ground black pepper

3 tablespoons dried parsley

Directions:

Preheat the oven to 400°F. Line a baking sheet with aluminum foil and spray with nonstick cooking spray.

In a mixing bowl, combine the mushrooms, garlic, avocado oil, Parmesan cheese, salt, and pepper. Mix well.

Spread the mushroom mixture on the prepared baking sheet and sprinkle with the parsley.

Bake for 12 minutes and stir. Return to the oven and bake for an additional 12 minutes.

Transfer the mushrooms to a serving dish.

Nutrition: Calories: 180 Cal Fat: 13 g

Protein: 8 g Carbs: 8 g Fiber: 1 g

75. Mediterranean Cucumber Bites

Preparation Time: 10 Minutes

Cooking Time: 0

Servings: 4

Ingredients:

8 ounces cream cheese, at room temperature

2 tablespoons chopped flat-leaf parsley

⅓ cup diced black olives

1 bell pepper, diced

2 cucumbers, halved lengthwise and seeded

2 tablespoons sliced scallions

Directions:

In a small bowl, mix together the cream cheese, parsley, olives, and bell pepper.

Fill each cucumber cavity with the cream cheese mixture. Sprinkle with the scallions, slice into 1-inch pieces, and serve.

Nutrition:

Calories: 253 Cal

Fat: 21 g

Protein: 6 g

Carbs: 10 g

Fiber: 2 g

Dinner Recipes

76. Seitan Tex-Mex Casserole

Preparation Time: 5 Minutes

Cooking Time: 35 Minutes

Servings: 4

Ingredients:

2 tbsp vegan butter

1 ½ lb seitan

3 tbsp Tex-Mex seasoning

2 tbsp chopped jalapeño peppers

½ cup crushed tomatoes

Salt and black pepper to taste

½ cup shredded vegan cheese

1 tbsp chopped fresh green onion to garnish

1 cup sour cream for serving

Directions:

Preheat the oven and grease a baking dish with cooking spray. Set aside.

Melt the vegan butter in a medium skillet over medium heat and cook the seitan until brown, 10 minutes.

Stir in the Tex-Mex seasoning, jalapeño peppers, and tomatoes; simmer for 5 minutes and adjust the taste with salt and black pepper.

Transfer and level the mixture in the baking dish. Top with the vegan cheese and bake in the upper rack of the oven for 15 to 20 minutes or until the cheese melts and is golden brown.

Remove the dish and garnish with the green onion.

Serve the casserole with sour cream.

Nutrition:

Calories: 464 Cal

Fat: 37.8 g

Carbs: 12 g

Fiber: 2 g

Protein: 24 g

77. Avocado Coconut Pie

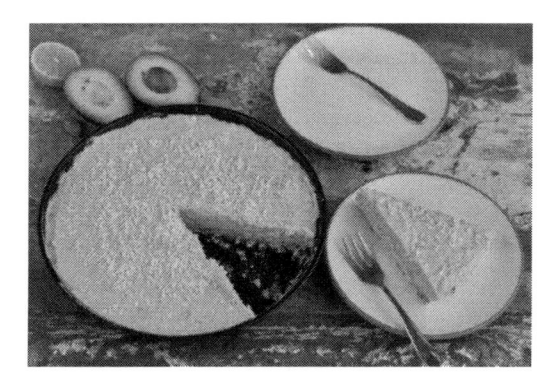

Preparation Time: 30 Minutes

Cooking Time: 50 Minutes

Servings: 4

Ingredients:

For the piecrust:

1 tbsp flax seed powder + 3 tbsp water

4 tbsp coconut flour

4 tbsp chia seeds

¾ cup almond flour

1 tbsp psyllium husk powder

1 tsp baking powder

1 pinch salt

3 tbsp coconut oil

4 tbsp water

For the filling:

2 ripe avocados

1 cup vegan mayonnaise

3 tbsp flax seed powder + 9 tbsp water

2 tbsp fresh parsley, finely chopped

1 jalapeno, finely chopped

½ tsp onion powder

¼ tsp salt

½ cup cashew cream

1¼ cups shredded tofu cheese

Directions:

In 2 separate bowls, mix the different portions of flax seed powder with the respective quantity of water. Allow absorbing for 5 minutes.

Preheat the oven to 350 F.

In a food processor, add the coconut flour, chia seeds, almond flour, psyllium husk powder, baking powder, salt, coconut oil, water, and the smaller portion of the flax egg. Blend the ingredients until the resulting dough forms into a ball.

Line a spring form pan with about 12-inch diameter of parchment paper and spread the dough in the pan. Bake for 10 to 15 minutes or until a light golden brown color is achieved.

Meanwhile, cut the avocado into halves lengthwise, remove the pit, and chop the pulp. Put in a bowl and add the mayonnaise, remaining flax egg, parsley, jalapeno, onion powder, salt, cashew cream, and tofu cheese. Combine well.

Remove the piecrust when ready and fill with the creamy mixture. Level the filling with a spatula and continue baking for 35 minutes or until lightly golden brown.

When ready, take out. Cool before slicing and serving with a baby spinach salad.

Nutrition:

Calories:680 Cal

Fat:71.8 g

Carbs: 10 g

Fiber:7 g

Protein: 3 g

78. Baked Mushrooms with Creamy Brussels Sprouts

Preparation Time: 8 Minutes

Cooking Time: 2 Hours 35 Minutes

Servings: 4

Ingredients:

For the mushrooms:

1 lb whole white button mushrooms

Salt and black pepper to taste

2 tsp dried thyme 1 bay leaf

5 black peppercorns

½ cups vegetable broth

2 garlic cloves, minced

1 ½ oz fresh ginger, grated

1 tbsp coconut oil   1 tbsp smoked paprika

For the creamy Brussel sprouts:

½ lb Brussel sprouts, halved

1 ½ cups cashew cream

Salt and ground black pepper to taste

Directions:

For the mushroom roast:

Preheat the oven to 200 F.

Pour all the mushroom ingredients into a baking dish, stir well, and cover with foil. Bake in the oven until softened, 1 to 2 hours.

Remove the dish, take off the foil, and use a slotted spoon to fetch the mushrooms onto serving plates. Set aside.

For the creamy Brussel sprouts:

Pour the broth in the baking dish into a medium pot and add the Brussel sprouts. Add about ½ cup of water if needed and cook for 7 to 10 minutes or until softened.

Stir in the cashew cream, adjust the taste with salt and black pepper, and simmer for 15 minutes.

Serve the creamy Brussel sprouts with the mushrooms.

Nutrition:

Calories: 492 Cal Fat: 37.9 g Carbs: 13 g

Fiber:2 g Protein: 29 g

79. Pimiento Tofu balls

Preparation Time: 10 Minutes

Cooking Time: 15 Minutes

Servings: 4

Ingredients: 1 tbsp Dijon mustard

¼ cup chopped pimientos

1/3 cup mayonnaise   3 tbsp cashew cream

1 tsp paprika powder

1 pinch cayenne pepper

4 oz grated vegan cheese

1 ½ lbs. tofu, pressed and crumbled

Salt and black pepper to taste

2 tbsp olive oil, for frying

Directions:

In a large bowl, add all the ingredients except for the olive oil and with gloves on your hands, mix the ingredients until well combined. Form bite size balls from the mixture.

Heat the olive oil in a medium non-stick skillet and fry the tofu balls in batches on both sides until brown and cooked through, 4 to 5 minutes on each side.

Transfer the tofu balls to a serving plate and serve warm.

Nutrition: Calories:254 Cal Fat: 36.8 g Carbs: 12 g Fiber: 1 g Protein:26 g

80. Tempeh with Garlic Asparagus

Preparation Time: 10 Minutes

Cooking Time: 18 Minutes

Servings: 4

Ingredients:

For the tempeh:

3 tbsp vegan butter

4 tempeh slices

Salt and black pepper to taste

For the garlic buttered asparagus:

2 tbsp. olive oil

2 garlic cloves, minced

1 lb asparagus, trimmed and halved

Salt and black pepper to taste

1 tbsp dried parsley

1 small lemon, juiced

Directions:

For the tempeh:

Melt the vegan butter in a medium skillet over medium heat, season the tempeh with salt, black pepper and fry in the butter on both sides until brown and cooked through, 10 minutes. Transfer to a plate and set aside in a warmer for serving.

For the garlic asparagus:

Heat the olive oil in a medium skillet over medium heat, and sauté the garlic until fragrant, 30 seconds.

Stir in the asparagus, season with salt and black pepper, and cook until slightly softened with a bit of crunch, 5 minutes.

Mix in the parsley, lemon juice, toss to coat well, and plate the asparagus.

Serve the asparagus warm with the tempeh.

Nutrition:

Calories: 181

Fat:17.5 g

Carbs: 6 g

Fiber: 3 g

Protein: 3 g

81. Mushroom Curry Pie

Preparation Time: 15 Minutes

Cooking Time: 55 Minutes

Servings 4

Ingredients:

For the piecrust:

1 tbsp flax seed powder + 3 tbsp water

¾ cup coconut flour

4 tbsp chia seeds

4 tbsp almond flour

1 tbsp psyllium husk powder

1 tsp baking powder

1 pinch salt

3 tbsp olive oil

4 tbsp water

For the filling:

1 cup chopped cremini mushrooms

1 cup vegan mayonnaise

3 tbsp + 9 tbsp water

½ red bell pepper, finely chopped

1 tsp turmeric powder

½ tsp paprika powder

½ tsp garlic powder

¼ tsp black pepper

½ cup cashew cream

1¼ cups shredded tofu cheese

Directions:

In two separate bowls, mix the different portions of flax seed powder with the respective quantity of water and set aside to absorb for 5 minutes.

Preheat the oven to 350 F.

Make the crust:

When the flax egg is ready, pour the smaller quantity into a food processor, add the coconut flour, chia seeds, almond flour, psyllium husk powder, baking powder, salt, olive oil, and water. Blend the ingredients until a ball forms out of the dough.

Line a springform pan with an 8-inch diameter parchment paper and grease the pan with cooking spray.

Spread the dough in the bottom of the pan and bake in the oven for 15 minutes.

Make the filling:

In a bowl, add the remaining flax egg, mushrooms, mayonnaise, water, bell pepper, turmeric, paprika, garlic powder, black pepper, cashew cream, and tofu cheese. Combine the mixture evenly and fill the piecrust. Bake further for 40 minutes or until the pie is golden brown.

Remove, slice, and serve the pie with a chilled strawberry drink.

Nutrition:

Calories:548 Cal

Fat: 55.9 g

Carbs: 6 g

Fiber: 2 g

Protein: 8 g

82. Spicy Cheese with Tofu Balls

Preparation Time: 20 Minutes

Cooking Time: 20 Minutes

Servings: 4

Ingredients:

For the spicy cheese:

1/3 cup vegan mayonnaise

¼ cup pickled jalapenos

1 tsp paprika powder

1 tbsp mustard powder

1 pinch cayenne pepper

4 oz grated tofu cheese

For the tofu balls:

1 tbsp flax seed powder + 3 tbsp water

2 ½ cup crumbled tofu

Salt and black pepper

2 tbsp plant butter, for frying

Directions:

Make the spicy cheese. In a bowl, mix the mayonnaise, jalapenos, paprika, mustard powder, cayenne powder, and cheddar cheese. Set aside.

In another medium bowl, combine the flax seed powder with water and allow absorbing for 5 minutes.

Add the flax egg to the cheese mixture, the crumbled tofu, salt, and black pepper, and combine well. Use your hands to form large meatballs out of the mix.

Then, melt the vegan butter in a large skillet over medium heat and fry the tofu balls until cooked and browned on the outside.

Serve the tofu balls with roasted cauliflower mash and mayonnaise.

Nutrition:

Calories: 259 Cal

Fat: 55.9 g

Carbs: 5 g

Fiber: 1 g

Protein: 16 g

83. Tempeh Coconut Curry Bake

Preparation Time: 7minutes

Cooking Time: 23minutes

Servings: 4

Ingredients:

1 oz. plant butter, for greasing

2 ½ cups chopped tempeh

Salt and black pepper

4 tbsp plant butter

2 tbsp red curry paste

1 ½ cup coconut cream

½ cup fresh parsley, chopped

15 oz. cauliflower, cut into florets

Directions:

Preheat the oven to 400 F and grease a baking dish with 1 ounce of vegan butter.

Arrange the tempeh in the baking dish, sprinkle with salt and black pepper, and top each tempeh with a slice of the remaining butter.

In a bowl, mix the red curry paste with the coconut cream and parsley. Pour the mixture over the tempeh.

Bake in the oven for 20 minutes or until the tempeh is cooked.

While baking, season the cauliflower with salt, place in a microwave-safe bowl, and sprinkle with some water. Steam in the microwave for 3 minutes or until the cauliflower is soft and tender within.

Remove the curry bake and serve with the caulis.

Nutrition:

Calories:417 Cal

Fat:38.8 g Carbs: 11 g

Fiber: 2 g

Protein: 11 g

84. Kale and Mushroom Pierogis

Preparation Time: 15 Minutes

Cooking Time: 30 Minutes

Servings: 4

Ingredients:

For the stuffing:

2 tbsp vegan butter

2 garlic cloves, finely chopped

1 small red onion, finely chopped

3 oz. baby bella mushrooms, sliced

2 oz. fresh kale

½ tsp salt   ¼ tsp black pepper

½ cup cashew cream   2 oz. grated tofu cheese

For the pierogi:

1 tbsp flax seed powder + 3 tbsp water

½ cup almond flour

4 tbsp coconut flour

½ tsp salt   1 tsp baking powder

1½ cups shredded tofu cheese

5 tbsp vegan butter

Olive oil for brushing

Directions:

Put the vegan butter in a skillet and melt over medium heat, then add and sauté the garlic, red onion, mushrooms, and kale until the mushrooms brown.

Season the mixture with salt and black pepper and reduce the heat to low. Stir in the cashew cream and tofu cheese and simmer for 1 minute. Turn the heat off and set the filling aside to cool.

Make the pierogis: In a small bowl, mix the flax seed powder with water and allow sitting for 5 minutes.

In a bowl, combine the almond flour, coconut flour, salt, and baking powder.

Put a small pan over low heat, add, and melt the tofu cheese and vegan butter while stirring continuously until smooth batter forms. Turn the heat off.

Pour the flax egg into the cream mixture, continue stirring, while adding the flour mixture until a firm dough form.

Mold the dough into four balls, place on a chopping board, and use a rolling pin to flatten each into ½ inch thin round pieces.

Spread a generous amount of stuffing on one-half of each dough, then fold over the filling, and seal the dough with your fingers.

Brush with olive oil, place on a baking sheet, and bake for 20 minutes or until the pierogis turn a golden-brown color.

Serve the pierogis with a lettuce tomato salad.

Nutrition: Calories:364

Fat:33.4 g Carbs:8g Fiber:2g Protein:12 g

85. Mushroom Lettuce Wraps

Preparation Time: 5minutes

Cooking Time: 16minutes

Servings: 4

Ingredients: 2 tbsp vegan butter

4 oz. baby bella mushrooms, sliced

1½ lbs. tofu, crumbled

½ tsp salt   ¼ tsp black pepper

1 iceberg lettuce, leaves extracted

1 cup shredded vegan cheese

1 large tomato, sliced

Directions:

Put the vegan butter in a skillet and melt over medium heat. Add the mushrooms and sauté until browned and tender, about 6 minutes. Transfer the mushrooms to a plate and set aside.

Add the tofu to the skillet, season with salt and black pepper, and cook until brown, about 10 minutes. Turn the heat off.

Spoon the tofu and mushrooms into the lettuce leaves, sprinkle with the vegan cheese, and share the tomato slices on top.

Serve the burger immediately.

Nutrition:

Calories:439 Cal Fat:31.9 g

Carbs: 9 g Fiber: 4 g Protein: 36 g

86. Tofu and Spinach Lasagna with Red Sauce

Preparation Time: 20 Minutes

Cooking Time: 45 Minutes

Servings: 4

Ingredients:

2 tbsp vegan butter

1 white onion, chopped

1 garlic clove, minced

2 ½ cups crumbled tofu

3 tbsp tomato paste

½ tbsp dried oregano

1 tsp salt

¼ tsp ground black pepper

½ cup water

1 cup baby spinach

Keto pasta

Flax egg: 8 tbsp flax seed powder + 1 ½ cups water

1 ½ cup dairy-free cashew cream

1 tsp salt

5 tbsp psyllium husk powder

Dairy-free cheese topping

2 cups coconut cream

5 oz. shredded vegan mozzarella cheese

2 oz. grated tofu cheese

½ tsp salt

¼ tsp ground black pepper

½ cup fresh parsley, finely chopped

Directions:

Melt the vegan butter in a medium pot over medium heat. Then, add the white onion and garlic, and sauté until fragrant and soft, about 3 minutes.

Stir in the tofu and cook until brown. Mix in the tomato paste, oregano, salt, and black pepper.

Pour the water into the pot, stir, and simmer the ingredients until most of the liquid has evaporated.

While cooking the sauce, make the lasagna sheets. Preheat the oven to 300 F and mix the flax seed powder with the water in a medium bowl to make flax egg. Allow sitting to thicken for 5 minutes.

Combine the flax egg with the cashew cream and salt. Add the psyllium husk powder a bit at a time while whisking and allow the mixture to sit for a few more minutes.

Line a baking sheet with parchment paper and spread the mixture in. Cover with another parchment paper and use a rolling pin to flatten the dough into the sheet.

Bake the batter in the oven for 10 to 12 minutes, remove after, take off the parchment papers, and slice the pasta into sheets that fit your baking dish.

In a bowl, combine the coconut cream and two-thirds of the mozzarella cheese. Fetch out 2 tablespoons of the mixture and reserve.

Mix in the tofu cheese, salt, black pepper, and parsley. Set aside.

Grease your baking dish with cooking spray, layer a single line of pasta in the dish, spread with some tomato sauce, 1/3 of the spinach, and ¼ of the coconut cream mixture. Season with salt and black pepper as desired.

Repeat layering the ingredients twice in the same manner making sure to top the final layer with the coconut cream mixture and the reserved cashew cream.

Bake in the oven for 30 minutes at 400 F or until the lasagna has a beautiful brown surface.

Remove the dish; allow cooling for a few minutes, and slice.

Serve the lasagna with a baby green salad.

Nutrition:

Calories:767 Cal

Fat: 69.8 g

Carbs:14g

Fiber: 3g

Protein: 28 g

87. Green Avocado Carbonara

Preparation Time: 15 Minutes

Cooking Time: 15 Minutes

Servings: 4

Ingredients:

8 tbsp flax seed powder + 1 ½ cups water

1 ½ cups dairy-free cashew cream

1 tsp salt

5 ½ tbsp psyllium husk powder

Avocado sauce

1 avocado, peeled and pitted

1 ¾ cups coconut cream

Juice of ½ lemon

1 teaspoon onion powder

½ teaspoon garlic powder

¼ cup olive oil

¾ teaspoon sea salt

¼ teaspoon black pepper

Walnut Parmesan or store-bought parmesan

For serving

4 tbsp toasted pecans

½ cup freshly grated tofu cheese

Directions:

Preheat the oven to 300 F.

In a medium bowl, mix the flax seed powder with water and allow sitting to thicken for 5 minutes.

Add the cashew cream, salt, and psyllium husk powder. Whisk until smooth batter forms.

Line a baking sheet with parchment paper, pour in the batter and cover with another parchment paper. Use a rolling pin to flatten the dough into the sheet.

Place in the oven and bake for 10 to 12 minutes. Remove the pasta after, take off the parchment papers and use a sharp knife to slice the pasta into thin strips lengthwise. Cut each piece into halves, pour into a bowl, and set aside.

For the avocado sauce, in a blender, combine the avocado, coconut cream, lemon juice, onion powder, and garlic powder. Puree the ingredients until smooth.

Pour the olive oil over the pasta and stir to coat properly. Pour the avocado sauce on top and mix. Then, season with salt, black pepper, and the soy cheese. Combine again.

Divide the pasta into serving plates, garnish with extra soy cheese and pecans, and serve immediately.

Nutrition:

Calories:941 Fat:94.2 g

Carbs:19 g Fiber:8 g

Protein:16g

88. Cashew Buttered Quesadillas with Leafy Greens

Preparation Time: 10 Minutes

Cooking Time: 20 Minutes

Servings: 4

Ingredients:

Tortillas

3 tbsp flax seed powder + ½ cup water

½ cup dairy-free cashew cream

1½ tsp psyllium husk powder

1 tbsp coconut flour

½ tsp salt

Filling

1 tbsp cashew butter, for frying

5 oz. grated vegan cheese

1 oz. leafy greens

Directions:

Preheat the oven to 400 F.

In a bowl, mix the flax seed powder with water and allow sitting to thicken for 5 minutes.

After, whisk the cashew cream into the flax egg until the batter is smooth.

In another bowl, combine the psyllium husk powder, coconut flour, and salt. Add the flour mixture to the flax egg batter and fold in until fully incorporated. Allow sitting for a few minutes.

Then, line a baking sheet with parchment paper and pour in the mixture. Spread into the baking sheet using a spatula and bake in the upper rack of the oven for 5 to 7 minutes or until brown around the edges. Keep a watchful eye on the tortillas to prevent burning.

Remove when ready and slice into 8 pieces. Set aside.

For the filling, spoon a little cashew butter into a skillet and place a tortilla in the pan. Sprinkle with some vegan cheese, leafy greens, and cover with another tortilla.

Brown each side of the quesadilla for 1 minute or until the cheese melts. Transfer to a plate.

Repeat assembling the quesadillas using the remaining cashew butter.

Serve immediately with avocado salad.

Nutrition:

Calories: 224 Cal

Fat: 20.4 g

Carbs: 1 g

Fiber: 0g

Protein: 9 g

89. Zucchini Boats with Vegan Cheese

Preparation Time: 3 Minutes

Cooking Time: 4 Minutes

Servings: 2

Ingredients:

1 medium-sized zucchini

4 tbsp vegan butter

2 garlic cloves, minced

1½ oz. baby kale

Salt and black pepper to taste

2 tbsp unsweetened tomato sauce

1 cup vegan cheese

Olive oil for drizzling

Directions:

Preheat the oven to 375 F.

Use a knife to slice the zucchini in halves and scoop out the pulp with a spoon into a plate. Keep the flesh.

Grease a baking sheet with cooking spray and place the zucchini boats on top.

Put the vegan butter in a skillet and melt over medium heat. Add and sauté the garlic until fragrant and slightly browned, about 4 minutes.

Add the kale and the zucchini pulp. Cook until the kale wilts; season with salt and black pepper.

Spoon the tomato sauce into the boats and spread to coat the bottom evenly. Then, spoon the kale mixture into the zucchinis and sprinkle with the cheese.

Bake in the oven for 20 to 25 minutes or until the cheese has a beautiful golden color.

Plate the zucchinis when ready, drizzle with olive oil, and season with salt and black pepper.

Serve immediately.

Nutrition:

Calories: 721 Cal Fat: 76.8 g

Carbs: 2 g Fiber: 0 g Protein: 9 g

90. Tempeh Garam Masala Bake

Preparation Time: 5 Minutes

Cooking Time: 24 Minutes

Servings: 4

Ingredients:

3 tbsp vegan butter

3 cups tempeh slices

Salt

2 tbsp garam masala

1 green bell pepper, finely diced

1¼ cups coconut cream

1 tbsp fresh cilantro, finely chopped

Directions:

Preheat the oven to 400 F.

Place a skillet over medium heat, add, and melt the vegan butter. Meanwhile, season the tempeh with some salt. Fry the tempeh in the butter until browned on both sides, about 4 minutes.

Stir half of the garam masala into the tempeh until evenly mixed; turn the heat off.

Transfer the tempeh with the spice into a baking dish.

Then, in a small bowl, mix the green bell pepper, coconut cream, cilantro, and remaining garam masala.

Pour the mixture over the tempeh and bake in the oven for 20 minutes or until golden brown on top.

Garnish with cilantro and serve with some cauli rice.

Nutrition:

Calories: 286 Cal

Fat: 27 g

Carbs: 5 g

Fibe r: 0 g

Protein: 9 g

91. Caprese Casserole

Preparation Time: 5 Minutes

Cooking Time: 20 Minutes

Servings: 4

Ingredients: 1 cup cherry tomatoes, halved

1 cup vegan mozzarella cheese, cut into small pieces

2 tbsp basil pesto

1 cup vegan mayonnaise

2 oz. tofu cheese

Salt and black pepper

1 cup arugula

4 tbsp olive oil

Directions:

Preheat the oven to 350 F.

In a baking dish, mix the cherry tomatoes, mozzarella, basil pesto, mayonnaise, half of the tofu cheese, salt, and black pepper.

Level the ingredients with a spatula and sprinkle the remaining tofu cheese on top. Bake for 20 minutes or until the top of the casserole is golden brown.

Remove and allow cooling for a few minutes. Slice and dish into plates, top with some arugula and drizzle with olive oil. Serve.

Nutrition: Calories: 588 Cal Fat: 59 g

Carbs: 2 g Fiber: 1 g Protein: 13 g

92. Lemon Garlic Mushrooms

Preparation Time: 25 Minutes

Cooking Time: 10 Minutes

Servings: 4

Ingredients: 3 oz enoki mushrooms

1 tbsp olive oil 1 tsp lemon zest, chopped

2 tbsp lemon juice

3 garlic cloves, sliced

6 oyster mushrooms, halved

5 oz cremini mushrooms, sliced

1/2 red chili, sliced

1/2 onion, sliced

1 tsp sea salt

Directions:

Heat olive oil in a pan over high heat.

Add shallots, enoki mushrooms, oyster mushrooms, cremini mushrooms, and chili.

Stir well and cook over medium-high heat for 10 minutes.

Add lemon zest and stir well. Season with lemon juice and salt and cook for 3-4 minutes.

Serve and enjoy.

Nutrition:

Calories: 87 Cal Fat: 5.6 gCarbs: 7.5 g

Sugar: 1.8 g Protein: 3 g

93. Almond Green Beans

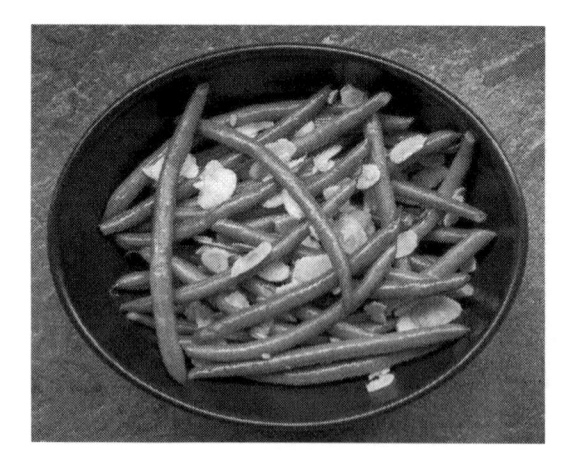

Preparation Time: 20 Minutes

Cooking Time: 5 Minutes

Servings: 4

Ingredients: ½ tsp sea salt

1 lb fresh green beans, trimmed

1/3 cup almonds, sliced 4 garlic cloves, sliced

2 tbsp olive oil 1 tbsp lemon juice

Directions:

Add green beans, salt, and lemon juice in a mixing bowl. Toss well and set aside. Heat oil in a pan over medium heat. Add sliced almonds and sauté until lightly browned. Add garlic and sauté for 30 seconds.

Pour almond mixture over green beans and toss well.

Stir well and serve immediately.

Nutrition: Calories: 146 Cal Fat: 11.2 g Carbs: 10.9 g Sugar: 2 g Protein: 4 g

94. Fried Okra

Preparation Time: 20 Minutes

Cooking Time: 5 Minutes

Servings: 4

Ingredients:

1 lb fresh okra, cut into ¼" slices

1/3 cup almond meal

Pepper

Salt

Oil for frying

Directions:

Heat oil in large pan over medium-high heat.

In a bowl, mix together sliced okra, almond meal, pepper, and salt until well coated.

Once the oil is hot then add okra to the hot oil and cook until lightly browned.

Remove fried okra from pan and allow to drain on paper towels.

Serve and enjoy.

Nutrition:

Calories: 91 Cal

Fat: 4.2 g

Carbs: 10.2 g

Sugar: 10.2 g

Protein: 3.9 g

95. Super Healthy Beet Greens Salad

Preparation Time: 10 Minutes

Cooking Time: 0

Servings: 4

Ingredients:

For Dressing:

1 garlic clove, minced

1 ½ teaspoons of dijon mustard

3 tablespoons of extra-virgin olive oil

1 tablespoon balsamic vinegar

Salt and freshly ground black pepper, to taste

2 cups of vegetable broth ¼ cup of olive oil

For Salad:

8 cup of fresh beet greens

¼ cup of feta cheese, crumbled

Directions:

Prepare dressing in a bowl by adding all the dressing ingredients and beat until well combined. In a large bowl, mix together greens and cheese.

Pour dressing over salad and toss to coat well. Serve immediately.

Nutrition:

Calories: 280   Fats: 26.2g   Carbs: 9.1g

Protein: 5.5g   Fiber: 3.6g

96. Coconut Yogurt with Chia Seeds and Almonds

Preparation Time: 10 Minutes

Cooking Time: 0

Servings: 4

Ingredients:

For Dressing:

1 1/3 cups of coconut yogurt

1 cup of unsweetened almond milk

8-10 drops of liquid stevia

Pinch of salt

1/3 cup of chia seeds

3 tablespoons of almonds, chopped

Directions:

In a bowl, add yogurt, milk, stevia, and salt and beat until well combined.

Add chia seeds and beat until well combined.

Refrigerate, covered for at least 4 hours.

Serve with a sprinkle of chopped almonds.

Nutrition:

Calories: 182 Cal

Fats: 9.1g

Carbs: 14.4g

Protein: 4.7g

Fiber: 10.8g

97. Super Delicious Cucumber Salad

Preparation Time: 10 Minutes

Cooking Time: 0

Servings: 8

Ingredients:

½ cup of sour cream

1 teaspoon of white vinegar

½ teaspoon of powdered stevia

½ teaspoon of dill weed

Salt, to taste

4 medium cucumbers, sliced

Directions:

In a bowl, add all the ingredients except cucumbers and beat until well combined.

Add cucumber slices and stir until well combined.

Refrigerate to chill for at least 30 minutes before serving.

Nutrition:

Calories: 54 Cal

Fats: 3.2g

Carbs: 6.1g

Protein: 1.4g

Fiber: 0.8g

98. Pudding Delight with Banana & Coconut

Preparation Time: 15 Minutes

Cooking Time: 0

Servings: 4

Ingredients:

1 medium banana, peeled and quartered

2 tablespoons of unsweetened coconut milk

1 packet of stevia

1 teaspoon of vanilla extract

1 cup of plain Greek yogurt

2 tablespoons of unsweetened coconut, shredded

Directions:

In a blender, add quartered bananas, milk, stevia, and vanilla extract and beat until well combined and smooth.

Transfer the mixture into a bowl.

Gently, fold in yogurt.

Refrigerate to chill completely.

Garnish with coconut and serve.

Nutrition:

Calories: 103 Cal   Fats: 4g

Carbs: 10.2g   Protein: 6.9g

Fiber: 1.2g

99. Extra Easy Cheese Sandwich

Preparation Time: 15 Minutes

Cooking Time: 5 Mins

Servings: 1

Ingredients:

2 tablespoons of almond flour

2 tablespoons of butter, softened

1½ tablespoons of psyllium husk powder

½ teaspoon of baking powder

2 large organic eggs

For Sandwiches:

2 tablespoons of cheddar cheese, grated

1 tablespoon of butter

Directions:

In a bowl, add all the bun ingredients except eggs and mix until a dough forms.

Add eggs and mix until a thick dough form.

Press each dough in a microwave safe square container.

Smooth the surface and clean of the sides.

Microwave for about 90-100 seconds.

Remove from microwave and keep aside to cool slightly.

Carefully remove the bun from container.

Cut the bun in half.

Place the cheese over cut side of 1 bun slices.

Cover with remaining bun slice to make a sandwich.

In a skillet, melt butter on medium heat.

Add sandwich and cook for about 1-2 minutes per side.

Nutrition:

Calories: 577 Cal Fats: 55.1g

Carbs: 4.7g Protein: 19g

Fiber: 1.6g

100. India Super Easy Summer Cooler

Preparation Time: 5 Minutes

Cooking Time: 0

Servings: 2

Ingredients:

1 cup of plain greek yogurt

1 cup of chilled water

Pinch of ground cumin

Pinch of paprika

Pinch of salt

Directions:

In a bowl, add yogurt and beat until smooth.

Slowly, add water, beating continuously.

Add spices and stir to combine well.

Pour into 2 serving glasses and serve immediately.

Nutrition:

Calories: 48 Cal

Fats: 1.3g

Carbs: 2.6g

Protein: 6.3g

Fiber: 0g

Dessert Recipes

101. Strawberry Coconut Parfait

Preparation Time: 5 Minutes

Cooking Time: 0

Servings: 4

Ingredients:

2 cups cold coconut yogurt

¼ cup fresh strawberries

½ lemon, zested

8 mint leaves

2 tbsp chia seeds

Maple (sugar-free) syrup to taste

Directions:

In four medium serving glasses, layer half of coconut yogurt, strawberries, lemon zest, mint leaves, chia seeds, and drizzle with maple syrup. Repeat with a second layer.

Serve.

Nutrition: Calories: 105 Cal

Fat: 7.82 g Carbs: 4.5 g

Fiber: 1.58 g

Protein: 5.24 g

102. Lemon-Chocolate Truffles

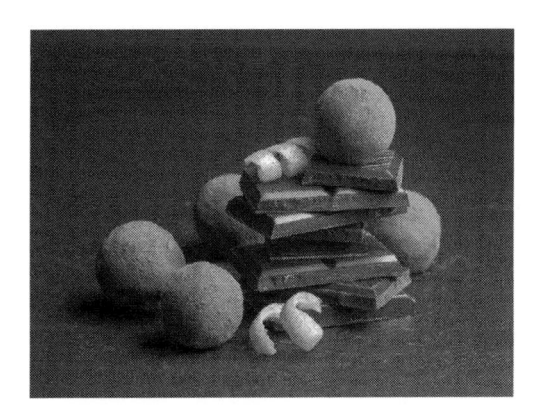

Preparation Time: 5 Minutes

Cooking Time: 30 Minutes

Servings: 4

Ingredients: 2/3 cup heavy cream

2/3 cup unsweetened dark chocolate, roughly chopped

½ lemon, juiced

¼ cup unsweetened cocoa powder

2 tbsp swerve sugar

Directions:

Over low fire, heat heavy cream in a small saucepan until tiny bubbles form around edges of pan. Turn heat off.

Add dark chocolate, swirl pan to coat chocolate with cream, and gently stir mixture until smooth.

Mix in lemon juice, pour mixture into a bowl, and chill for 4 hours or until mixture hardens for molding.

Line two baking trays with parchment papers; set one aside and mix cocoa powder and swerve sugar in other.

Remove chocolate mixture from fridge; form bite-size balls and coat in cocoa powder.

Place truffles on other baking tray and chill for 30 minutes before serving.

Nutrition:

Calories: 143 Cal Fat: 12.68 g

Carbs: 3.13 g Fiber: 2.5 g Protein: 2.41 g

103. Blackberry and Red Wine Crumble

Preparation Time: 10 Minutes

Cooking Time: 45 Minutes

Servings: 6

Ingredients:

2 cups blackberries

¼ cup red wine

1 tsp cinnamon powder

1 tsp vanilla extract

1 ¼ cup erythritol, divided

1 cup cold salted butter, cubed

¾ cup coconut flour

1 ½ cups almond flour

Directions:

Preheat oven to 375o F.

In a baking dish, add blackberries, red wine, cinnamon powder, vanilla, half of erythritol, and stir.

In a medium bowl, using your hands, rub butter with coconut flour, almond flour, and remaining erythritol until resembles large breadcrumbs.

Spread mixture over blackberries making sure to cover well; bake until golden brown on top, 45 minutes.

Remove from oven; allow cooling for 3 minutes and serve warm.

Nutrition:

Calories: 318 Cal

Fat: 31.34 g

Carbs: 9.79 g

Fiber: 4.9 g

Protein: 1.5 g

104. Cinnamon-Chocolate Cake

Preparation Time: 20 Minutes

Cooking Time: 45 Minutes

Servings: 4

Ingredients: ½ cup melted butter

1 cup almond flour

½ cup unsweetened dark chocolate, melted

1 cup erythritol 2 tsp vanilla caviar

½ tsp salt 2 tsp cinnamon powder

½ cup boiling water 3 large eggs

Swerve confectioner's sugar for garnishing

Directions:

Preheat oven to 350oF, lightly grease a springform pan with cooking spray and line with parchment paper. Set aside.

In a large bowl, mix butter, almond flour, chocolate, erythritol, vanilla, salt, cinnamon powder, and boiling water. Crack eggs one after another while continually beating until smooth. Pour batter into springform pan and bake in oven until a toothpick inserted comes out clean, 45 minutes.

Remove from oven; allow cooling in pan for 10 minutes and turn over onto a wire rack.

Dust with swerve confectioner's sugar, slice, and serve.

Nutrition: Calories: 417 Cal Fat: 41.75 g

Carbs: 11.53 g Fiber: 9.8 g Protein: 16.45 g

105. Himalayan Raspberry Fat Bombs

Preparation Time: 15 Minutes

Cooking Time: 0

Servings: 4

Ingredients:

3 cups golden Himalayan raspberries

1 tsp vanilla extract

16 oz cream cheese, room temperature

4 tbsp unsalted butter

2 tbsp maple (sugar-free) syrup

Directions:

Line a 12-holed muffin tray with cake liners and set aside.

Pour raspberries, vanilla into a blender, and puree until smooth.

In a small saucepan, over medium heat, melt cream cheese and butter until well-combined.

In a medium bowl, evenly combine raspberry mix, cream cheese mix, and maple syrup. Pour mixture into muffin holes.

Refrigerate for 40 minutes and serve after.

Nutrition:

Calories: 227 g Fat: 14.8 g

Carbs: 5.2 g Fiber: 2.1 g Protein: 4.68 g

106. Cashew-Chocolate Cheesecake

Preparation Time: 10 Minutes

Cooking Time: 6 Minutes

Servings: 4

Ingredients:

For crust:

1 cup raw cashew nuts

½ cup salted butter, melted

2 tbsp swerve sugar

For cake:

1 tsp agar powder

2 tbsp lemon juice

2/3 cup unsweetened dark chocolate, chopped + extra for garnishing

4 tbsp unsalted butter, melted

1 ½ cups cream cheese

½ cup erythritol

1 cup Greek yogurt

Directions:

For crust:

Preheat oven to 350oF.

In a food processor, blend cashews until finely ground. Add butter, swerve sugar, and mix until combined.

Press crust mixture firmly into bottom of a spring form pan.

Bake for 5 minutes and chill while you prepare the filling.

For cake:

In a small pot, combine agar with lemon juice, and a tablespoon of water. Allow sitting for 5 minutes and then, set pot over medium heat to dissolve agar. Set aside.

In a medium safe-microwave bowl, add dark chocolate, butter, and microwave for 1 minute to melt, stirring at every 10 seconds interval. Set aside.

In another medium bowl, beat cream cheese with erythritol until smooth. Stir in agar and yogurt until evenly combined. Fold in chocolate and mix well.

Remove pan from fridge and pour cream mixture on top. Tap sides of pan gently to release trapped air bubbles; transfer pan to fridge and chill for at least 3 hours.

When ready, remove and release cake from pan, garnish with dark chocolate, and slice.

Serve immediately.

Nutrition:

Calories: 235 Cal

Fat: 14.12 g

Carbs: 7.3 g

Fiber: 3.5 g Protein: 6.78 g

107. Creamy Avocado Drink

Preparation Time: 5 Minutes

Cooking Time: 0

Servings: 4

Ingredients:

4 large ripe avocados, halved and pitted

1 tsp vanilla extract

4 tbsp erythritol

¼ cup cold unsweetened almond milk

1 tbsp cold heavy cream

Directions:

In a blender, add avocado pulp, vanilla extract, erythritol, almond milk, and heavy cream. Process until smooth.

Pour mixture into serving glasses and serve immediately.

Nutrition:

Calories: 388 Cal

Fat: 32.16 g

Carbs: 5.42 g

Fiber: 3.32 g

Protein: 6.95 g

108. Raspberry Cookies

Preparation Time: 10 Minutes

Cooking Time: 25 Minutes

Servings: 6

Ingredients: 1 tablespoon ground flaxseed

1 cup blanched almond flour

2 tablespoon coconut flour

1 cup granulated Swerve

1/2 cup almond butter

1/8 teaspoon vanilla extract

1/4 cup almond milk 1/2 cup raspberries

1/4 cup sugar-free chocolate chips

Directions: Mix ground flaxseed with 2.5 tablespoon water in a bowl and keep it aside for 10 minutes. Let your oven preheat at 350 degrees F then layer an 8-inch pan with parchment paper. IN a bowl whisk all the dry ingredients then stir in almond butter, milk, vanilla extracts, and flaxseed mixture. Mix well until combined, add few drops of more milk if the mixture is too thick. Fold in half of the chocolate and raspberries to the batter. Spread this raspberry batter in the layered pan evenly then top it with remaining raspberries and chocolate chips. Bake the batter for 25 minutes until golden brown. Slice and serve fresh.

Nutrition: Calories: 234 Cal

Fat: 17.3 g Carbs: 6.9 g Protein: 4.8 g

109. Lenny & Larry's Cookies

Preparation Time: 10 Minutes

Cooking Time: 10 Minutes

Servings: 6

Ingredients:

3 tablespoon coconut flour

1 scoop vanilla protein powder

2 tablespoon nut butter

1 tablespoon swerve

1-2 tablespoon almond milk

Directions:

Let your oven preheat at 350 degrees F and layer a baking tray with parchment paper.

Whisk everything dry in a bowl first then stir in wet ingredients.

Mix well until it forms crumbly mixture then add some liquid to make a thick batter.

Make small dough balls out of this mixture and place them in the baking tray.

Press the balls with the palm of your hand to make flat cookies.

Bake them for 10 minutes then serve.

Nutrition:

Calories: 206 Cal

Fat: 20.3 g Carbs: 2.6 g

Protein: 4.2 g

110. Zucchini Chocolate Brownies

Preparation Time: 10 Minutes

Cooking Time: 25 Minutes

Servings: 6

Ingredients: 1/3 cup coconut oil

1 1/4 cups chocolate chips

3/4 cup granulated Swerve

1/4 cup zucchini, grated   2 large eggs

2 tablespoon cocoa powder

3 tablespoon arrowroot powder

Directions:

Let your oven preheat at 350 degrees F. Layer an 8-inch pan with parchment sheet and grease it with cooking oil.

Melt and mix chocolate with coconut oil in a bowl by heating in the microwave for 30 seconds. Whisk this mixture with eggs, sweetener, and zucchini. Stir in arrowroot powder and cocoa powder. Mix well until smooth.

Spread this mixture in the pan evenly then bake it for 25 minutes until done. Allow it to cool for 15 minutes then slice.

Enjoy fresh.

Nutrition:

Calories: 280 Cal Fat: 23 g

Carbs: 3.1 g Protein: 3.9 g

111. Fudgy Pumpkin Brownies

Preparation Time: 10 Minutes

Cooking Time: 35 Minutes

Servings: 4

Ingredients: 4 eggs

1 cup pumpkin puree 1 cup mashed avocado

2 cups of cocoa powder

6 tablespoon coconut flour

2/3 cup swerve

1 tablespoon baking soda

1 cup unsweetened coconut milk

1/2 cup sugar-free chocolate chips

Directions:

Let your oven preheat at 350 degrees F. Layer an 8-inch pan with parchment paper. On high speed blend everything in a food processor except chocolate chips and coconut milk. Once mix well then add ½ cup coconut milk and continue mixing. Add more coconut milk if the mixture is too thick. Spread this batter evenly in the layered pan and sprinkle chocolate chips over the batter. Bake the batter for 35 minutes until golden brown.

Slice and serve fresh.

Nutrition:

Calories: 211 Cal Fat: 26 g

Carbs: 3.1 g Protein: 3.9 g

112. Cinnamon Roll Bars

Preparation Time: 10 Minutes

Cooking Time: 0

Servings: 6

Ingredients: 3/4 cup coconut flour

2 cups cashew butter   1/2 cup swerve

1 1/2 tablespoon cinnamon divided

8 oz cream cheese, softened

1/4 cup granulated Swerve

Directions:

Layer an 8-inch pan with parchment paper then keep it aside.

Mix smooth nut butter, coconut flour and a tablespoon of cinnamon in a bowl to make a thick batter.

Add some more liquid if the mixture is too thick then transfer this mixture to a pan.

Spread this mixture evenly and refrigerate for a few hours.

Meanwhile, beat cream cheese with sweetener and half tablespoon cinnamon.

Spread this mixture over the refrigerate batter evenly. Slice the base into 12 equal-sized bars.

Serve fresh.

Nutrition:

Calories: 166 Cal Fat : 25.5 g Carbs: 5.5 g

Protein: 4.9 g

113. Snickers Bars

Preparation Time: 10 Minutes

Cooking Time: 1 Minute

Servings: 6

Ingredients: 1.5 cups almond butter

1 cup salted nuts   1/2 cup nut or seed butter

3/4 cup coconut flour

2 cups almond butter   1/2 cup swerve

1 teaspoon water 1-2 tablespoon almond milk

1-2 cups sugar-free chocolate chips

Directions:

Blend almond butter with nuts in a food processor on high speed to make a thick paste.

Spread this mixture in an 8-inch pan, lined with parchment paper and refrigerate.

Prepare the caramel by heating seed butter, coconut oil, and swerve in a pan.

Pour this mixture in the pan and freeze again until firm. Slice the base into small-sized bars.

Melt chocolate in a bowl by heating in the microwave for a 1 minute. Dip the bars in the melted chocolate and refrigerate them until chocolate is set. Enjoy fresh.

Nutrition:

Calories: 181 Cal Fat: 14.7 g

Carbs: 7.4 g Protein: 6.3 g

114. Lemon Coconut Crack Bars

Preparation Time: 10 Minutes

Cooking Time: 0

Servings: 6

Ingredients:

3 cups unsweetened shredded coconut

1-2 tablespoon lemon rind, chopped

1/3 cup coconut oil

3/4 cup swerve

Directions:

Toss everything into a large mixing bowl and mix well until combined.

Layer an 8-inch pan with parchment paper.

Spread the prepared batter in the pan evenly and firmly.

Place the pan in the freezer then slice the batter into small bars.

Enjoy fresh.

Nutrition:

Calories: 149 Cal

Fat: 15.1 g

Carbs: 5.1 g

Protein: 0.8 g

115. Gingerbread Cookie Bars

Preparation Time: 10 Minutes

Cooking Time:

Servings: 6

Ingredients: 2 cups cashew butter

1/2 cup swerve 3/4 cup coconut flour

1 teaspoon nutmeg 2 teaspoon ground ginger

1 teaspoon cinnamon

1 serving cream cheese

Directions:

Melt and mix cashew butter with sweetener in a bowl by heating in the microwave for 30 seconds.

Start adding the remaining ingredients and mix well to form a thick batter.

Layer an 8-inch square pan with parchment paper.

Spread the prepared batter in the pan evenly and firmly. Refrigerate for 4 hours.

Slice into small bars and top them with cream cheese.

Refrigerate again for 30 minutes.

Enjoy.

Nutrition:

Calories: 103 Cal Fat: 12.3 g

Carbs: 8.4 g Protein: 3.1g

116. Cocoa Berries Mousse

Preparation Time: 10 Minutes

Cooking Time: 0

Servings: 2

Ingredients:

1 tablespoon cocoa powder

1 cup blackberries

1 cup blueberries

¾ cup coconut cream

1 tablespoon stevia

Directions:

In a blender, combine the berries with the cocoa and the other ingredients, pulse well, divide into bowls and keep in the fridge for 2 hours before serving.

Nutrition:

Calories: 200 Cal

Fat: 8 g

Fiber: 3.4 g

Carbs: 7.6 g

Protein: 4.3 g

117. Nutmeg Pudding

Preparation Time: 10 Minutes

Cooking Time: 20 Minutes

Servings: 6

Ingredients:

2 tablespoons stevia

1 teaspoon nutmeg, ground

1 cup cauliflower rice

2 tablespoons flaxseed mixed with 3 tablespoons water

2 cups almond milk

¼ teaspoon nutmeg, grated

Directions:

In a pan, combine the cauliflower rice with the flaxseed mix and the other ingredients, whisk, cook over medium heat for 20 minutes, divide into bowls and serve cold.

Nutrition:

Calories: 220 Cal

Fat: 6.6 g

Fib er: 3.4 g

Carbs: 12.4 g

Protein: 3.4 g

118. Lime Cherries and Rice Pudding

Preparation Time: 10 Minutes

Cooking Time: 25 Minutes

Servings: 4

Ingredients:

¾ cup stevia

2 cups coconut milk

3 tablespoons flaxseed mixed with 4 tablespoons water

Juice of 2 limes

Zest of 1 lime, grated

1 cup cherries, pitted and halved

1 cup cauliflower rice

Directions:

In a pan, combine the milk with the stevia and bring to a simmer over medium heat.

Add the cauliflower rice and the other ingredients, stir, cook for 25 minutes more, divide into cups and serve cold.

Nutrition:

Calories: 199 Cal

Fat: 5.4 g

Fiber: 3.4 g Carbs: 11g

Protein: 5.6 g

119. Chocolate Pudding

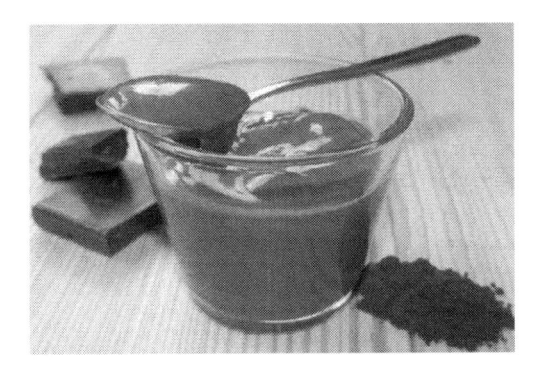

Preparation Time: 10 Minutes

Cooking Time: 20 Minutes

Servings: 4

Ingredients: 2 tablespoons cocoa powder

2 tablespoons coconut oil, melted

2/3 cup coconut cream

2 tablespoons stevia

¼ teaspoon almond extract

Directions:

In a pan, combine the cocoa powder with the coconut milk and the other ingredients, whisk, bring to a simmer ad cook over medium heat for 20 minutes.

Divide into cups and serve cold.

Nutrition:

Calories: 134 Cal Fat: 14.1 g

Fiber: 0.8 g Carbs: 3.1 g

Protein: 0.9 g

120. Coffee and Rhubarb Cream

Preparation Time: 10 Minutes

Cooking Time: 20 Minutes

Servings: 4

Ingredients:

¼ cup brewed coffee

2 tablespoons stevia

2 cups coconut cream

1 teaspoon vanilla extract

2 tablespoons coconut oil, melted

1 cup rhubarb, chopped

2 tablespoons flaxseed mixed with 3 tablespoons water

Directions:

In a bowl, mix the coffee with stevia, cream and the other ingredients, whisk well and divide into 4 ramekins.

Introduce the ramekins in the oven at 350 degrees F, bake for 20 minutes and serve warm.

Nutrition:

Calories: 300 Cal

Fat: 30.8 g

Fiber: 0 g

Carbs: 3 g

Protein: 4 g

121. Chocolate Sea Salt Almonds

Preparation Time: 10 Minutes

Cooking Time: 0

Servings: 8

Ingredients:

4 ounces low-carb chocolate, chopped

1 tablespoon coconut oil

1 cup dry-roasted almonds

Sea salt

Directions:

Line a rimmed baking sheet with parchment paper.

In a small saucepan over medium-low heat, melt the chocolate and coconut oil together while stirring constantly. Remove from the heat once melted and pour into a small bowl.

Add the almonds to the chocolate and give them a good stir.

Using a teaspoon, remove a cluster of almonds and place it on the prepared baking sheet. Immediately sprinkle with a bit of sea salt.

Repeat step 4 with the remaining nuts.

Place the baking sheet in the refrigerator for 30 minutes or until set.

Remove and store the clusters in small resealable plastic bags (or cover each cluster with plastic wrap) in the refrigerator until ready to eat.

Nutrition:

Calories: 187 Cal Fat: 15 g

Protein: 6 g Carbs: 7 g Fiber: 4 g

122. Salted Caramel Cashew Brittle

Preparation Time: 10 Minutes

Cook Time: 5 Minutes

Servings: 6

Ingredients:

8 tablespoons grass-fed butter

4 tablespoons brown erythritol, granulated

4 ounces raw unsalted cashews

4 tablespoons natural cashew butter

Coarse sea salt

Directions:

Line a rimmed baking sheet with parchment paper.

In a small saucepan over low heat, stir the butter until it melts.

Add the erythritol, cashews, and cashew butter. Mix until thoroughly combined and melted.

Pour the mixture onto the prepared baking sheet.

Sprinkle salt on top.

Place the baking sheet in the refrigerator to harden for about 1 hour.

Remove the brittle from the sheet and break into about 12 pieces.

Nutrition:

Calories: 321 Cal Fat: 29 g

Protein: 5 g Carbs: 10 gFiber: 1 g

123. Cookies and Cream Parfait

Preparation Time: 5 Minutes

Cooking Time: 0

Servings: 1

Ingredients:

½ scoop low-carb vanilla protein powder

¾ cup plain full-fat Greek yogurt

1 Oreo cookie

4 tablespoons sugar-free chocolate syrup (I like Walden Farms)

Directions:

In a small bowl, mix together the protein powder and Greek yogurt until smooth and creamy.

Remove one side of the Oreo cookie. Place it in a small resealable plastic bag and crush it with the back of a spoon. Set aside.

Pour the chocolate syrup over the yogurt mixture and sprinkle with the cookie crumbles.

Nutrition:

Calories: 281 Cal Fat: 13 g Protein: 19 g

Carbs: 22 g Fiber: 3 g

124. Pecan Pie Pudding

Preparation Time: 5 Minutes

Cooking Time: 0

Servings: 1

Ingredients:

¾ cup plain full-fat Greek yogurt

½ scoop low-carb vanilla protein powder

4 tablespoons chopped pecans

2 tablespoons sugar-free syrup

Directions:

In a small bowl, mix together the Greek yogurt and protein powder until smooth and creamy.

Top with the chopped pecans and syrup.

Nutrition: Calories: 381 Cal Fat: 21 g

Protein: 32 gCarbs: 16 gFiber: 7 g

125. Chocolate Avocado Pudding

Preparation Time: 5 Minutes

Cooking Time: 0

Servings: 1

Ingredients:

1 avocado, halved

⅓ cup full-fat coconut milk

1 teaspoon vanilla extract

2 tablespoons unsweetened cocoa powder

5 or 6 drops liquid stevia

Directions:

Combine all the ingredients in a high-powered blender or food processor and blend until smooth. Serve immediately.

Nutrition:

Calories: 555 Cal

Fat: 47 g

Protein: 7 g

Carbs: 26 g

Fiber: 17 g

Conclusion

The Ketogenic diet is truly life changing. The diet improves your overall health and helps you lose the extra weight in a matter of days. The diet will show its multiple benefits even from the beginning and it will become your new lifestyle really soon.

As soon as you embrace the Ketogenic diet, you will start to live a completely new life. On the other hand, the vegetarian diet is such a healthy dietary option you can choose when trying to live healthy and also lose some weight.

The collection we bring to you today is actually a combination between the Ketogenic and vegetarian diets. You get to discover some amazing Ketogenic vegetarian dishes you can prepare in the comfort of your own home. All the dishes you found here follow both the Ketogenic and the vegetarian rules, they all taste delicious and rich and they are all easy to make.

You have already made the lifestyle decision to eat vegetarian foods, now add to that decision the choice to eat a keto lifestyle. By adding these two lifestyle choices together you will have the two most powerful weapons for weight loss and healthy living at your disposal. You now possess all the knowledge that you need in order to make this new lifestyle change to keto vegetarianism.

The different herbs and spices that were featured in this book have shown you how easy it is to create tasty dishes. You have recipes for many different sauces that will help to compliment your vegetarian choices without totally blowing your keto diet plan. You have recipes for delicious breakfasts, lunches, and dinners. We showed you how to create a sample meal plan that will teach you how easy it is to make good choices when it comes to the food that you put in your body. And we even gave you some recipes for desserts because we know you are human and life is so much better when it includes a little treat every now and then.

Most importantly we hope you now see that living the keto vegetarian lifestyle is not impossible. It might not be one of the easiest things you will ever do but it will enrich your life and your health far beyond anything you might ever have imagined.

We can assure you that such a combo is hard to find. So, start a keto diet with a vegetarian "touch" today. It will be both useful and fun!

So, what are you still waiting for? Get started with the Ketogenic diet and learn how to prepare the best and most flavored Ketogenic vegetarian dishes. Enjoy them all!

Printed in Great Britain
by Amazon